Respiratory and Airway Emergencies

Editors

HANEY MALLEMAT
TERREN TROTT

EMERGENCY MEDICINE CLINICS OF NORTH AMERICA

www.emed.theclinics.com

Consulting Editor
AMAL MATTU

August 2022 • Volume 40 • Number 3

ELSEVIER

1600 John F. Kennedy Boulevard • Suite 1800 • Philadelphia, Pennsylvania, 19103-2899

http://www.theclinics.com

EMERGENCY MEDICINE CLINICS OF NORTH AMERICA Volume 40, Number 3
August 2022 ISSN 0733-8627, ISBN-13: 978-0-323-98709-7

Editor: Joanna Collett

Developmental Editor: Axell Ivan Jade Purificacion

Emergency Medicine Clinics of North America (ISSN 0733-8627) is published quarterly by Elsevier Inc., 360 Park Avenue South, New York, NY, 10010-1710. Months of issue are February, May, August, and November. Business and Editorial Offices: 1600 John F. Kennedy Boulevard, Suite 1800, Philadelphia, PA 19103-2899. Customer Service Office: 6277 Sea Harbor Drive, Orlando, FL 32887-4800. Periodicals postage paid at New York, NY, and additional mailing offices. Subscription prices are $100.00 per year (US students), $370.00 per year (US individuals), $963.00 per year (US institutions), $220.00 per year (international students), $476.00 per year (international individuals), $1002.00 per year (international institutions), $100.00 per year (Canadian students), $436.00 per year (Canadian individuals), and $1002.00 per year (Canadian institutions). International air speed delivery is included in all *Clinics'* subscription prices. All prices are subject to change without notice. **POSTMASTER:** Send address changes to *Emergency Medicine Clinics of North America*, Elsevier Periodicals Customer Service, 11830 Westline Industrial Drive, St. Louis, MO 63146. Customer Service (orders, claims, online, change of address): Elsevier Periodicals **Customer Service, 11830 Westline Industrial Drive, St. Louis, MO 63146. Tel: 1-800-654-2452 (U.S. and Canada); 314-453-7041 (outside U.S. and Canada). Fax: 314-453-5170. E-mail: journalscustomerservice-usa@elsevier.com (for print support);** journalsonlinesupport-usa@elsevier.com **(for online support).**

Reprints. For copies of 100 or more of articles in this publication, please contact the Commercial Reprints Department, Elsevier Inc., 360 Park Avenue South, New York, NY 10010-1710. Tel.: 212-633-3874; Fax: 212-633-3820; E-mail: reprints@elsevier.com.

Emergency Medicine Clinics of North America is covered in *MEDLINE/PubMed (Index Medicus), Current Contents/Clinical Medicine, EMBASE/Excerpta Medica, BIOSIS, SciSearch, CINAHL, ISI/BIOMED,* and *Research Alert.*

Contributors

CONSULTING EDITOR

AMAL MATTU, MD, FAAEM, FACEP
Professor and Vice Chair of Academic Affairs, Department of Emergency Medicine, University of Maryland School of Medicine, Baltimore, Maryland

EDITORS

HANEY MALLEMAT, MD
Associate Professor, Department of Internal Medicine and Emergency Medicine, Emergency Medicine/Critical Care Medicine Program, Cooper Medical School at Rowan University, Cooper University of Rowan University, Camden, New Jersey

TERREN TROTT, MD
Assistant Professor, Departments of Pulmonary, Critical Care and Sleep Medicine and Emergency Medicine, University of Kentucky, Lexington, Kentucky

AUTHORS

JASON BOWMAN, MD
Department of Pulmonary, Critical Care and Sleep Medicine, University of Kentucky, Lexington, Kentucky

KENNETH BUTLER, DO
Associate Professor of Emergency Medicine, Associate Residency Director, Department of Emergency Medicine, University of Maryland School of Medicine, Baltimore, Maryland

SARA E. CRAGER, MD
Assistant Professor, Departments of Emergency Medicine and Critical Care Anesthesia, University of California, Los Angeles, Los Angeles, California

HARMAN S. GILL, MD
Assistant Professor, Departments of Emergency Medicine, and Medicine, Section of Pulmonary and Critical Care Medicine, Dartmouth Geisel School of Medicine

ALIN GRAGOSSIAN, DO, MPH
Department of Critical Care Medicine, The Mount Sinai Hospital, New York, New York

DUNCAN GROSSMAN, DO
Assistant Professor, Department of Emergency Medicine, The Mount Sinai Hospital, New York, New York

MAX HOCKSTEIN, MD
Departments of Emergency Medicine and Critical Care, MedStar Washington Hospital Center

CAROLINE HUMPHREYS, MD
Department of Emergency Medicine, University of California, Los Angeles, Los Angeles, California

LAUREN A. IGNERI, PharmD, BCPS, BCCCP
Clinical Pharmacy Specialist, Critical Care, Department of Pharmacy, Cooper University Healthcare, Camden, New Jersey

BRIT LONG, MD
Associate Professor of Military and Emergency Medicine, SAUSHEC, Brooke Army Medical Center, Fort Sam Houston, Texas

HANEY MALLEMAT, MD
Associate Professor, Department of Internal Medicine and Emergency Medicine, Emergency Medicine/Critical Care Medicine Program, Cooper Medical School at Rowan University, Cooper University of Rowan University, Camden, New Jersey

EVIE G. MARCOLINI, MD
Associate Professor, Departments of Emergency Medicine and Neurology, Division of Neurocritical Care, Geisel School of Medicine at Dartmouth

CHRISTOPHER NOEL, MD
Division of Critical Care, Cooper University Health Care, Cooper Medical School of Rowan University, Cooper University Hospital, Camden, New Jersey

BRIAN C. PARK, MD
Critical Care Medicine Program, Cooper University of Rowan University, Camden, New Jersy

RACHEL RAFEQ, PharmD
PGY2 Residency Program Director, Clinical Pharmacy Specialist, Emergency Medicine, Department of Pharmacy, Cooper University Healthcare, Camden, New Jersey

SALIM R. REZAIE, MD
Greater San Antonio Emergency Physicians (GSEP), Director of Clinical Education, Associate Clinical Professor, University of the Incarnate Word School of Osteopathic Medicine, Previous Editor in Chief of *Emergency Physicians Monthly*, Medical Director of IA MED, Emergency Medicine/Internal Medicine, Creator/Founder of REBEL EM (www.rebelem.com)

MATTHEW T. SIUBA, DO
Department of Critical Care Medicine, Respiratory Institute, Cleveland Clinic, Cleveland, Ohio

BRANDON SOMWARU, DO
Department of Emergency Medicine, St. Joseph's University Medical Center, Paterson, New Jersey

RORY SPIEGEL, MD
Departments of Emergency Medicine, and Critical Care, MedStar Washington Hospital Center

TERREN TROTT, MD
Assistant Professor, Departments of Pulmonary, Critical Care and Sleep Medicine and Emergency Medicine, University of Kentucky, Lexington, Kentucky

JARED WARD, DO, MPH
Critical Care, Inspira Health Network, Inspira Medical Center Vineland, Vineland, New
Jersey

MICHAEL WINTERS, MD, MBA, FACEP, FAAEM
Professor of Emergency Medicine and Medicine, Vice Chair for Clinical and Administrative
Affairs, Department of Emergency Medicine, University of Maryland School of Medicine,
Baltimore, Maryland

Contents

Emergency clinicians are tasked with managing a variety of patients with acute deformities. One of the most acute situations management of the patient who presents with an airway emergency. Patients present with various pathologies may result in anatomically challenging intubation scenarios. Deferral of intubation is often not an option in the emergency department. In some cases, challenging anatomic issues can be predicted before beginning laryngoscopy, but in many situations, prediction models fall short. It is critically important for emergency clinicians to anticipate anatomic issues in all airways and to have premeditated strategies for managing them.

Acute respiratory distress syndrome (ARDS) occurs in up to 10% of patients with respiratory failure admitted through the emergency department. Use of noninvasive respiratory support has proliferated in recent years; clinicians must understand the relative merits and risks of these technologies and know how to recognize signs of failure. The cornerstone of ARDS care of the mechanically ventilated patient is low-tidal volume ventilation based on ideal body weight. Adjunctive therapies, such as prone positioning and neuromuscular blockade, may have a role in the emergency department management of ARDS depending on patient and department characteristics.

Acute respiratory failure requiring invasive mechanical ventilation is a common presentation in the emergency department. Providers can further improve care for these patients by understanding common modes of mechanical ventilation, recognizing changes in respiratory mechanics, and tailoring ventilator settings and therapies accordingly.

Airway pressure release ventilation (APRV) is a mode of ventilation that uses high airway pressures to recruit and maintain patients' lung volumes. The goal of this mode of ventilation is 2-fold: first, to maintain patients as close to their functional residual capacity as possible and second, to promote safe spontaneous breathing. APRV should essentially be viewed as continuous positive airway pressure (CPAP), with intermittent releases of that pressure to metabolically support patients who are incapable of managing their ventilatory load. As patients recruit and lungs approach the patients' natural lung volumes, their ability to breathe spontaneously and manage their own ventilatory needs improves. Eventually, patients are able to fully support their ventilatory needs and no longer require any release breaths to maintain normal CO_2 levels. Now, patients can be "stretched" to CPAP.

Pneumonia is a lower respiratory tract infection caused by the inability to clear pathogens from the lower airway and alveoli. Cytokines and local inflammatory markers are released, causing further damage to the lungs through the accumulation of white blood cells and fluid congestion, leading to pus in the parenchyma. The Infectious Diseases Society of America defines pneumonia as the presence of new lung infiltrate with other clinical evidence supporting infection, including new fever, purulent sputum, leukocytosis, and decline in oxygenation. Importantly, lower respiratory infections remain the most deadly communicable disease. Pneumonia is subdivided into three categories: (1) community acquired, (2) hospital acquired, and (3) ventilator associated. Therapy for each differs based on the severity of the disease and the presence of risk factors for methicillin-resistant Staphylococcus aureus or Pseudomonas aeruginosa.

Right ventricular dysfunction is an important component of the pathophysiology of several disorders commonly encountered in the emergency department (ED). Interventions often performed routinely early in the ED course such as fluid administration and endotracheal intubation have the potential to cause precipitous clinical deterioration in patients with right ventricular failure and pulmonary hypertension. It is important for emergency physicians to understand the pathophysiology of acute decompensated right ventricular failure in order to avoid common pitfalls in diagnosis and management that can result in significant morbidity and mortality.

Obstructive lung disease includes asthma and chronic obstructive pulmonary disease (COPD). Exacerbation of asthma or COPD can result in significant morbidity and mortality, and emergency department (ED) care is often required. ED evaluation should assess risk factors for severe exacerbation and the patient's hemodynamic and respiratory status. Assessments including chest radiograph, point-of-care ultrasound, capnography, and electrocardiogram can assist. First-line treatments for acute exacerbation include bronchodilators and corticosteroids. Noninvasive ventilation, magnesium, ketamine, and epinephrine should be considered in those with severe exacerbation. Mechanical ventilation is challenging and should use an obstructive lung strategy with permissive hypercapnia.

Pulmonary embolism is a challenging pathology commonly faced by emergency physicians, and diagnosis and management remain a crucial skill set. Inherent to the challenge is the breadth of presentation, ranging from asymptomatic pulmonary emboli to sudden cardiac death. Diagnosis and exclusion have evolved over time and now use a combination of clinical decision calculators and updates to the classic d-dimer cutoffs. Management of pulmonary emboli revolves around appropriate anticoagulation, which for most of the patients will comprise newer oral agents. However, there remains a substantial degree of practice variation and ambiguity when it comes to higher risk patients with submassive or massive pulmonary emboli.

In the emergency department, there are infrequent but essential procedures related to pulmonary diseases that emergency physicians must be able to perform. These include thoracentesis, chest tube thoracostomy, tracheostomy manipulation, and fiberoptic intubation.

This article explains the physiologic basis and fundamentals behind the technology of continuous positive airway pressure, bilevel positive airway pressure, and high flow nasal canula. Additionally, it explores some of the core literature behind their clinical applications. It will also compare HFNC with other noninvasive modalities for respiratory failure alongside clinical titration and weaning algorithms in the emergency department setting.

Emergency physicians intubate critically ill patients almost daily. Intubation of the critically ill emergency department (ED) patient is a high-risk, high-stress situation, as many have physiologic derangements such as hypotension, hypoxemia, acidosis, and right ventricular dysfunction that markedly increase the risk of peri-intubation cardiovascular collapse and cardiac arrest. This chapter discusses critical pearls and pitfalls to intubate the critically ill ED patient with physiologic derangements. These pearls and pitfalls include appropriate preoxygenation; circulatory resuscitation; proper patient position and room setup; selection of medications for rapid sequence intubation; and intubation of patients with severe acidosis, traumatic brain injury, and pulmonary hypertension.

EMERGENCY MEDICINE CLINICS OF NORTH AMERICA

SERIES OF RELATED INTEREST

Critical Care Clinics
https://www.criticalcare.theclinics.com/
Chest Medicine
https://www.chestmed.theclinics.com/

THE CLINICS ARE NOW AVAILABLE ONLINE!
Access your subscription at:
www.theclinics.com

Foreword
Pulmonary Emergencies

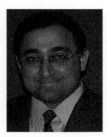

Amal Mattu MD, FAAEM, FACEP
Consulting Editor

The mantra of emergency medicine is "A-B-C," airway, breath sounds, circulation, and it is no surprise why. These represent the fastest causes of death—loss of airway, inadequate breathing, and compromised circulation—and consequently they represent the first priorities in resuscitation. It is noteworthy that two of these three components focus on the respiratory status of the patient. Loss of airway function and compromise of lung function are the most rapid killers in emergency medicine, and so it is appropriate that they receive the first and foremost attention in acute resuscitation. Quite simply, if a provider possesses clinical excellence with the "A" and the "B," then lives are saved. Conversely, if a provider lacks skills in the "A" and the "B," then patients die…very quickly.

In this issue of *Emergency Medicine Clinics of North America*, critical care experts Drs Haney Mallemat and Terren Trott have brought together a panel of experts in resuscitation to advance our skills in the management of airway and respiratory emergencies. Articles focus on both basic and advanced airway management techniques and challenges. Articles also focus on the challenge of managing patients on ventilators. Ventilatory management in past decades has been of lesser importance for emergency physicians, but with increased emergency department boarding this past decade, it has become more important than ever for us to know basic as well as advanced ventilatory management, and these articles fit the bill perfectly.

The authors also address specific high-risk diseases, including right ventricular failure, pulmonary infections, pulmonary embolism, and reactive airway disease. A separate article also focuses on special procedures for patients with pulmonary disease.

This issue of *Emergency Medicine Clinics of North America* is a must-read for every emergency physician. Regardless of years of experience, readers will find life-saving pearls and learn practice-changing tips to improve patient care on a daily basis. Our

Emerg Med Clin N Am 40 (2022) xiii–xiv
https://doi.org/10.1016/j.emc.2022.06.002
0733-8627/22/© 2022 Published by Elsevier Inc.

emed.theclinics.com

sincerest thanks go to Dr Mallemat, Dr Trott, and their outstanding set of authors for providing this amazing resource to us all.

Amal Mattu, MD, FAAEM, FACEP
Department of Emergency Medicine
University of Maryland School of Medicine
110 South Paca Street
6th Floor, Suite 200
Baltimore, MD 21201, USA

E-mail address:
amattu@som.umaryland.edu

Preface

Airways and Breathing in Emergency Medicine

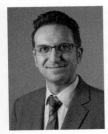 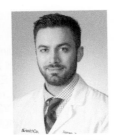

Haney Mallemat, MD   Terren Trott, MD
Editors

Emergency Medicine physicians are tasked with caring for some of the most critically ill patients who enter the hospital. They must rapidly stabilize and manage patients with septic shock, cardiac arrest, and major trauma. One of the most challenging issues Emergency Physicians face is airway management and respiratory diseases. Inability to manage a patient's airway may rapidly lead to death or disability. Respiratory diseases alone or in combination with airway management can also lead to a rapid decline in a patient's clinical status and worsen outcomes.

In this issue of *Emergency Medicine Clinics of North America*, our authors tackle some of the fundamental topics in airway management and respiratory disease. These core topics are ubiquitous in the field of emergency medicine and remain challenging topics in management despite advances in our medical understanding. Some topics reviewed include high-intensity high-stakes presentations that require premediated review and even rehearsal of management. These represent some of our sickest patients, such as the crashing asthmatic or patient with a massive pulmonary embolism. Alternatively, we discuss the approach to our difficult airways, whether those be a bleeding necrotic neck cancer or the intubation of a patient with a pH of 6.7 and a respiratory rate of 44. Our authors navigate these challenging patients, and subsequent articles outline ventilator management and troubleshooting.

How do we approach the patient who appears to be fighting the ventilator to the point of hypoxia? Refractory hypoxia and hypercapnia are reviewed in articles on airway-pressure release ventilation, noninvasive ventilation, acute respiratory distress syndrome, and ventilator dyssynchrony. Adjuncts to management and special procedures are reviewed, such as chest tube placement and fiberoptic intubation. Past initial stabilization and initiation of mechanical ventilation, we also review core topics, such as management of respiratory infections, chronic obstructive pulmonary disease,

Emerg Med Clin N Am 40 (2022) xv–xvi
https://doi.org/10.1016/j.emc.2022.06.001
0733-8627/22/© 2022 Published by Elsevier Inc.

and pulmonary hypertension. These topics, combined, highlight the challenge and importance of airway management and respiratory disease by Emergency Medicine.

Haney Mallemat, MD
Department of Internal Medicine and
Emergency Medicine
Cooper Medical School at Rowan University
1 Cooper Medical Plaza
Camden, NJ 08103, USA

Terren Trott, MD
Department of Pulmonary, Critical Care
and Sleep Medicine and
Emergency Medicine
University of Kentucky
222 Arlington Avenue
Lexington, KY 40508, USA

E-mail addresses:
haney.mallemat@gmail.com (H. Mallemat)
terren.trott@gmail.com (T. Trott)

Intubating Special Populations

Brandon Somwaru, DO[a],*, Duncan Grossman, DO[b],1

KEYWORDS

- Difficult airway • Neck trauma • Airway contamination • Burns • Angioedema
- Anaphylaxis

KEY POINTS

- Several patient groups present anatomically challenging airways. These airways can be difficult to predict making it critical that the emergency clinicians have a structured approach to managing them when they arise.
- Prehospital and emergency department management of cervical spine injuries, whether present or suspected, presents a barrier to endotracheal tube delivery. It is important to understand techniques to minimize injury while maximizing the success of intubation.
- Dynamic airways, those with rapidly progressive anatomic issues, are uncommon but present unique challenges. These include anaphylaxis, angioedema, and penetrating neck wounds. Rapid airway control is often indicated in these pathologies.
- Pregnant patients may have challenging airway management from a gravid uterus as well as physiologic tissue changes secondary to hormonal changes.
- Patients with obesity are at high risk of desaturation and may benefit from specific techniques to optimize positioning and preoxygenation.

INTRODUCTION

Patients with anatomically challenging airways can present enormous barriers to the delivery of an endotracheal tube. These challenges include both structural abnormalities and deformities that alter or obscure the airway anatomy. Extensive evidence shows that it is extremely difficult to predict which patients will have a challenging airway anatomy despite the presence of numerous tools designed for this purpose.[1] As a result of this limitation, preparation for a challenging airway scenario should be the default approach to all emergency airway scenarios. Despite the limitations of prediction instruments, there are certain patient features that should prompt the

[a] Department of Emergency Medicine, St. Joseph's University Medical Center, 703 Main Street, Paterson, NJ, 07503, USA; [b] Department of Emergency Medicine, The Mount Sinai Hospital, New York, NY, USA
[1] Present address: 40 Wildwood Avenue, West Orange, NJ 07052.
* Corresponding author. 703 Main Street, Paterson, NJ, 07503.
E-mail address: brandon.somwaru1@gmail.com

Emerg Med Clin N Am 40 (2022) 443–458
https://doi.org/10.1016/j.emc.2022.05.001
0733-8627/22/© 2022 Elsevier Inc. All rights reserved.

emed.theclinics.com

emergency clinician to expect specific challenges. These patient groups include, but are not limited to, those with suspected cervical spine injuries or abnormalities, dynamic airways (anaphylaxis, expanding hematomas, or infections), pregnancy, obesity, head and neck cancers, facial fractures, trismus, and those with airway contamination or potential for contamination.

Airway Decontamination

The presence of blood, mucus, emesis, or foreign materials in the airway can create immense challenges in the delivery of an endotracheal tube. Airway soiling impedes direct visualization of the vocal cords and can complicate video laryngoscopy (VL) techniques by coating the camera lens rendering the device ineffective. Contamination can result from several pathologies including excessive secretions (ie, cholinergic toxidrome), hemorrhage (ie, gastrointestinal, resulting from trauma, postoperative, pulmonary), and vomitus.

Consider the placement of a nasogastric tube (NGT) before intubation. NGT placement can empty the stomach and decrease the risk of large-volume aspiration and airway contamination. As such, an NGT will only benefit if the source of contamination is gastrointestinal (ie, GI bleeding or vomitus). If the patient is unable to tolerate NGT placement but it is determined to be of benefit, ketamine can be used to facilitate placement followed by intubation (ie, delayed sequence intubation [DSI]).

Preoxygenation is important before intubation but should be applied safely. If the patient requires bag-valve-mask (BVM) ventilation, a positive end-expiratory pressure (PEEP) valve should be used. Target a PEEP of less than 20 cm H2O to prevent opening of the lower esophageal sphincter, gastric insufflation, and increased risk of emesis.[2]

Patient positioning can help to reduce airway contamination as well. Elevate the head of the bed to 45° to aid in reducing the risk of gastric contents filling the hypopharynx and mouth. This is particularly helpful if the contaminant is the result of gastrointestinal hemorrhage or vomitus. Keeping the patient semi-upright may also improve preoxygenation by decreasing the collapse of both upper airway soft tissues and lower airway alveoli. Although the "bed-up-head-elevated" (BUHE) positioning (**Fig. 1**) has been shown to improve safe apnea times and first-pass success and decrease intubation-related complications in the anesthesia literature, no difference has been found in first-pass success among ED intubations in limited studies.[3–6]

Airway contamination will occasionally occur despite best efforts at prevention. The most commonly used device for airway decontamination is the Yankauer suction catheter. Although this device can provide effective clearing in circumstances of light secretions or small amounts of blood, it is ill-equipped to clear significant soilage. The suction tip of the Yankauer is narrow providing a low level of suction as well as the inability to suction anything except for fluids. This results from the fact that the Yankauer was developed to provide gentle suction for Otolaryngologist in the operating room.

Recently, larger bore suction catheters have emerged. These devices have larger diameters allowing them to effectively suction blood (both fresh and clotted) as well as vomitus making them clearly superior devices. Although having the proper equipment is important, decontamination technique is vital as well. Suction-Assisted Laryngoscopy for Airway Decontamination is a technique developed by Dr Jim DuCanto which allows the airway operator to effectively manage patients with significant airway contamination. If used prophylactically, it may decrease the risk of contamination.[7] Please refer to the following video for a demonstration of the technique (https://spaces.hightail.com/receive/V0YyRzYPqP). The steps are summarized in **Box 1** (see **Fig. 1** for technique description).

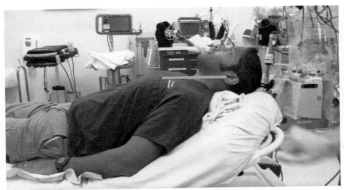

Fig. 1. Bed-up-head-elevated (BUHE) positioning. Intubating clinicians may find that they too need to be elevated to manage the airway of a patient in the BUHE position. This can be achieved by dropping the stretcher to its lowest position, getting a small step (typically used for chest compressions), or even standing on the back frame of the stretcher. (Photo Courtesy of Anand Swaminathan, MD.)

Dynamic Airways

Introduction

Dynamic airway processes pose a nuanced challenge to airway management. We define the dynamic airway as one in which the underlying deformities may cause rapid deterioration of airway patency. This process can convert a patent airway into a cannot intubate, cannot oxygenate (CICO) scenario in minutes forcing the clinician to perform a surgical airway. The dynamic airway category includes, but is not limited to, inhalation injuries/airway burns, penetrating neck trauma, and anaphylaxis/angioedema. Each of these scenarios forces the clinician to weigh the need for early definitive

---

Box 1
Suction-assisted laryngoscopy for airway decontamination technique

1. Lead with a rigid suction catheter (held in the right hand) and suction any proximal airway contaminant

2. Insert the video laryngoscope into the midline of the mouth (with left hand)

3. Continue to advance the suction catheter followed by the laryngoscope. The suction catheter not only clears the airway of any blood, vomitus, or other secretions but also helps to lift the tongue

4. Place the laryngoscope in the vallecula and visualize the vocal cords

5. Move and "park" the suction catheter to the left corner of the mouth, with the tip of the catheter in the proximal esophagus. The catheter can then be pinned in place by the laryngoscope in the left hand, resulting in continuous esophageal suctioning with endotracheal tube insertion on the right. If available, an assistant can also hold the suction catheter in place as laryngoscopy occurs.

6. Advance the endotracheal tube through the vocal cords. Secure and suction the tube.

Source: Suction Assisted Laryngoscopy and Airway Decontamination (SALAD). https://www.sscor.com/suction-assisted-laryngoscopy-and-airway-decontamination-salad. Accessed November 30, 2019.

airway management before deterioration versus the risk that definitive airway management is not necessary, along with the harm of waiting to manage the airway only to have deterioration occur.

Burns and inhalation injuries

Inhalation injuries are frequently classified by location, either above or below the glottis. Supraglottic injuries are commonly caused by thermal burns, whereas subglottic injuries are often caused by noxious chemicals present in smoke. Thermal burns typically affect the upper airway given the respiratory tract's ability to exchange heat whereas irritant gases affect the lower airway by eliciting local tissue inflammation and epithelial damage.[8,9]

Traditional teaching for patients with inhalation injuries stresses early intubation because concerns that inflammation, in combination with fluid resuscitation, could cause soft tissue edema. Extensive soft tissue edema could lead to distorted airway anatomy or airway obstruction and often prompts early intervention. The American Burn Association's relative indications for early intubation are listed in **Box 2**.

Although early intubation can be a lifesaving procedure, several retrospective studies suggest that more than 30% of burn patients are intubated unnecessarily.[10–12] Unnecessary intubation poses several risks such as avoidable transfers, ventilator-related complications, and death. Unfortunately, data supporting specific well validated criteria for early intubation are inconsistent. Several studies dispute the accuracy of physical findings, such as singed nasal or facial hair.[13]

Inhalation injuries severe enough to require intubation can be diagnosed by fiberoptic bronchoscopy. However, this resource is unavailable in many emergency departments. As an alternative, clinicians can use the Denver criteria listed in **Box 3**. A 2018 retrospective review of intubated burn patients led to the creation of the Denver criteria, which was shown to be more sensitive, but less specific than traditional teaching and American Burn Association (ABA) guidelines (see **Box 3**).[14] VL and point-of-care ultrasound may also be useful in predicting airway injury, although additional data are needed.[15,16]

Anaphylaxis and angioedema

Anaphylaxis and angioedema are distinct diseases but both syndromes can cause severe soft tissue swelling and possible airway obstruction.

Like all dynamic airways, airway patency during anaphylaxis or angioedema can change rapidly. Airways previously determined to be patent can deteriorate and

---

Box 2
Relative indications for early intubation[8]

Stridor

Dysphonia

Accessory muscle use

Large burns involve greater than 40 to 50% TBSA

Deep facial burns

Intraoral burns

Difficulty swallowing

Inability to clear secretions

Concerns for progressive airway edema during transport if patient requires transfer

| Box 3 |
Denver criteria[14]
Full-thickness facial burns
Stridor
Respiratory distress
Swelling on laryngoscopy
Upper airway trauma
Altered mentation
Hypoxia/hypercarbia
Hemodynamic instability
Suspected smoke inhalation
Hoarseness
Dysphagia
Singed facial hair
Non-full-thickness facial burn

physicians should monitor patients closely for changes that may indicate impending airway compromise. These signs and symptoms include voice changes, hoarseness, dyspnea, and stridor.[17] Although patients with isolated facial, lip, and soft palate edema rarely require airway intervention, the risk of intubation increases as edema extends posteriorly to the tongue and larynx.[6] Frequent assessments of the posterior oropharynx can help guide treatment and determine the need for intervention.

Prompt and aggressive treatment of anaphylaxis and angioedema diseases can reduce the need of intubation. Early administration of icatibant, ecallantide, and recombinant c1 inhibitor may prevent worsening of symptoms in patients with bradykinin-mediated angioedema secondary to hereditary C1 inhibitor deficiency. With respect to anaphylaxis, early administration of epinephrine can reduce the risk of intubation by decreasing mucosal edema.[18,19] Although intramuscular epinephrine is recommended as first-line, nebulized epinephrine can be considered in the setting of upper airway obstruction.[7] For patients with persistent worrisome symptoms after epinephrine administration, early intubation should be considered.

Penetrating neck trauma

The spectrum of severity in patients with penetrating neck trauma ranges from patients who can be safely discharged to traumatic arrest due to airway compromise. The nature of injuries and their locations can vary widely; thus, it is difficult to make standardized recommendations for this heterogenous group of injuries.

Penetrating neck injuries may lead to airway compromise through two main mechanisms. First, the airway itself may be injured. This can impair the mechanics of breathing and lead to further obstruction of the airway with blood or foreign bodies. Second, injury to the structures in the neck surrounding the airway may be injured and lead to distortion of the anatomy thus jeopardizing the airway. This includes vascular injury leading to an expanding hematoma compressing the airway as well as massive subcutaneous air causing airway distortion. Penetrating neck injuries are often dynamic in nature, and a patent airway may become unstable during a trauma resuscitation.

The decision to intubate a patient may depend not only on their clinical status but on their expected course. Patients may benefit from early intubation if they have dynamic airway features (ie, expanding hematoma) or if they are going directly to the operating room.

General recommendations for dynamic airways

Owing to the inherent challenges associated with dynamic airways, we endorse several universal intubation principles to aid in successful airway management. These general recommendations include preparing multiple airway approaches with a range of devices and techniques, the use of fiberoptic laryngoscopy when available, and awake intubation if appropriate. Listed below are specific recommendations as they apply to each distinct dynamic airway deformities.

Burns and inhalation injuries specific recommendations

Fiberoptic laryngoscopy remains the preferred strategy for intubating burn patients by virtue of its ability to serve as both a diagnostic and therapeutic modality. Clinicians using fiberoptic laryngoscopy will be able to access the extent and depth of the burn while also safely securing the airway.

Contrary to popular belief, depolarizing paralytic agents, such as succinylcholine, can be used early in burn care. The risk of hyperkalemia is caused by the release of potassium from upregulated extrajunctional acetylcholine receptors. This phenomenon occurs 24 to 72 h post-injury and can persist for up to 1 year.[20]

In addition, the ABA recommends using a cuffed endotracheal tube with a diameter large enough to facilitate aggressive pulmonary toileting and diagnostic or therapeutic bronchoscopy.[7]

Anaphylaxis/angioedema specific recommendations

Like inhalation injuries, fiberoptic laryngoscopy remains beneficial for intubating patients with anaphylaxis and angioedema. Expert recommendations favor a fiberoptic-guided nasotracheal approach as it can help physicians navigate more skillfully around obstructions while reducing inadvertent airway complications from excessive manipulation.[21] A relatively large prospective multicenter cohort study evaluating patients with angioedema showed that fiberoptic laryngoscopy was the most successful intubation technique when compared with rigid VL and direct laryngoscopy (DL).[22] In addition, nasotracheal attempts using fiberoptic laryngoscopy were more successful than those performed via the orotracheal route.[22]

Awake intubation should also be considered for patients with anaphylaxis or angioedema. Consensus statements advise against rapid sequence intubation (RSI) when angioedema is so severe that the upper airway cannot be directly visualized.[21] Avoiding sedative and paralytic agents preserves intrinsic respiratory function and has been associated with higher rates of success in patients with angioedema.[22] Topical anesthesia with or without sedative medications can help facilitate awake intubation in patients with impending airway instability with multiple studies showing topical anesthesia to be equal or superior to sedative medications, including ketamine.[23]

Once again, early intubation should be considered in this patient population to prevent CICO scenarios.

Penetrating neck trauma-specific recommendations

The ideal approach to intubation of patients with penetrating neck injuries is unknown. The Eastern Association for the Surgery of Trauma (EAST) stated the same in 2012 and advocated for DL or awake nasotracheal intubation as the preferred approach. However, none of the studies cited for these recommendations evaluated VL.[24] An awake or ketamine-facilitated approach may be beneficial as they allow the patient to continue breathing spontaneously and maintain airway architecture that can be lost when paralytics are administered.

Traditional RSI has been shown to be reasonable and effective in these patients.[25] In 2018, the Royal College of Surgeons of England recommended RSI for patients with intact anatomy, and fiberoptic intubation for patients in whom the airway anatomy may be disrupted.[26]

Obesity

Patients with obesity pose unique challenges during airway management, although their classification as a "difficult airway" is vague and requires clarification. A patient may have a difficult airway because of difficult laryngoscopy, difficult intubation, or other difficult airway maneuvers that do not involve intubation at all. These patients often have limited neck mobility, redundant airway tissue, altered pharmacokinetics, and other features that complicate multiple facets of airway management. However, the literature regarding the intubation of patients with obesity is conflicting with several studies suggesting that body mass index (BMI) is not a reliable predictor of difficult endotracheal intubation (ETI).[27–29]

Adequate preoxygenation of patients with obesity is essential when preparing to perform ETI. Patients with obesity desaturate much more quickly than leaner patients after induction for several reasons. The mass of the chest can compress the thoracic cavity, and substantial abdominal viscera may further restrict lung inflation and alveolar recruitment, particularly in the supine position. In addition, patients with obesity have a higher baseline metabolism and consume oxygen at a faster rate than leaner patients.[23] BVM ventilation can be extremely difficult if the intubation is unsuccessful.[30] Positioning the patient upright during preoxygenation has been shown to increase safe apneic times.[4] Using noninvasive positive pressure ventilation at 100% FiO_2 as a preoxygenation method has been shown to delay time to desaturation by up to 60 s.[31]

Positioning the patient before induction (do you mean the patient or ETI; this statement is unclear) is essential in this patient group, as it may be difficult to position them after induction or in the setting of a failed intubation attempt when there is difficulty with reoxygenating.

Awake, flexible endoscopic intubation is more commonly performed in the morbidly obese population by anesthesiologists and may be an appropriate, safe method.[32] If the patient is amenable to this approach, nasotracheal intubation via flexible endoscopy can be performed with the patient seated upright. However, this technique requires practice, experience, adequate topicalization, special equipment, and a cooperative patient.

For patients who will undergo conventional RSI, DSI, or sedation-only procedures, intubating these patients in the BUHE position may be advantageous. As mentioned above, the supine position creates problematic physiology in patients with obesity; thus, maintaining an upright position throughout the procedure may be beneficial. The BUHE position has been associated with improved laryngoscopy views, even in patients without obesity.[33] This position also prolongs the amount of time it takes for patients with obesity to desaturate during intubation.[23] To place a patient in the BUHE position, the operator should raise the head of the bed to 25° and position the head so the external auditory meatus is parallel to the sternal notch (see **Fig. 1**).

In the event of a failed airway, as mentioned previously, clinicians may have a particularly difficult time using a BVM to reoxygenate patients with obesity. A supraglottic device must be readily available at the bedside when intubating a patient with obesity and should be incorporated into the airway plan. Some of these devices will allow clinicians to intubate through them (with flexible endoscopy or a tracheal tube introducer) and may be of particular benefit in the event of an unanticipated difficult laryngoscopy or intubation.

For the failed intubation, cricothyrotomy may be necessary but poses its challenges due to redundant tissue and difficulty palpating landmarks. Before performing ETI, clinicians should consider palpating for landmarks and mark the midline of the neck with a surgical marker. However, these landmarks may be difficult to palpate in the patient with obesity. Ultrasound has been shown to be a fast and effective way to identify the cricothyroid membranes in these patients and may help with marking the anatomy.[34]

Pregnancy

Acute respiratory failure is an uncommon presentation in pregnancy, occurring in only approximately one in 500 pregnant or postpartum patients.[35] However, despite its relative infrequency, respiratory failure has particularly devastating consequences in this patient population if not managed appropriately. Although clinicians should prioritize treating the underlying etiology of the patient's respiratory failure, intubation may be required for stabilization or definitive management. Unfortunately, limited data regarding emergency airway intervention in pregnant people are available. Nevertheless, understanding the changes that occur in pregnancy can help facilitate successful intubation and airway management.

Causes of respiratory failure in pregnant people include those specific to pregnancy, those exacerbated by pregnancy, and those found within the general population (**Table 1**).[3]

Regardless of the cause, emergency clinicians must be aware of the anatomic and physiologic changes that make airway management challenging.

Airway anatomy in pregnant people is affected by numerous changes, including hormones secreted during gestation. Human placental growth factor can make soft tissue more edematous and friable, leading to an increased risk of airway edema and bleeding.[36] Clinicians should consider these risks when choosing laryngoscopy type and endotracheal tube size to maximize first-pass success and prevent iatrogenic obstruction.

A gravid abdomen, large breast tissue, and pregnancy-associated obesity can further complicate airway management. These changes can distort airway anatomy and impede correct pre-intubation positioning, proper BVM seal, or lead to aortocaval compression.[37] Uterine displacement, achieved by a left lateral tilt of 15° or manual displacement of the uterus with the patient fully supine, can prevent aortocaval

Table 1
Pathologies associated with pregnancy[4]

Pathologies Specific to Pregnancy	Pathologies with Increased Risk in Pregnancy	Pathologies Common in the General Population
Preeclampsia	Veno-thromboembolism	Nonobstetric sepsis
Eclampsia	Aspiration	Trauma
Obstetric sepsis	Asthma	Drugs/toxins
Peripartum cardiomyopathy	Heart failure	
Amniotic fluid embolism	Transfusion-related acute lung injury	
	Gastric acid aspiration	

compression and reduce the risk of hemodynamic collapse.[38] Depending on the clinical scenario, a fluid bolus to increase preload volume before intubation may be warranted to mitigate the risk of peri-intubation hypotension.

If contemplating intubation in a peripartum patient, clinicians should reassess airway anatomy frequently. A small prospective study indicated that traditional tools used by anesthesia to predict difficult airways, such as the Mallampati score, change not only throughout pregnancy but also during labor.[39]

Physiologic changes secondary to the various anatomic changes also increase the risk of a difficult airway. A gravid uterus decreases functional residual capacity (FRC) by 10% to 25%, whereas oxygen consumption increases by 20% to 33% by the third trimester due to increased metabolic demands from the fetus.[31] Increased oxygen consumption, in combination with decreased FRC and basilar atelectasis, can cause rapid peri-intubation oxygen desaturation. Aggressive preoxygenation and denitrogenation, followed by apneic oxygenation, can delay desaturations during laryngoscopy.

Hormone-mediated changes not only affect airway anatomy but also gastrointestinal tract physiology. Progesterone decreases lower esophageal sphincter tone, which can lead to gastric contents entering the airway during intubation. Clinicians should also avoid bag-mask ventilation if possible to prevent gastric overdistention. Intubating with the head of the bed elevated at 30° (BUHE) may decrease aspiration risk while simultaneously improving apneic oxygenation by relieving uterine compression of the lung bases and increasing FRC (see **Fig. 1**).[40]

Head and Neck Cancers

With more than 550,000 new cases a year, head and neck cancers continue to contribute to approximately 3% of all cancers worldwide.[41] In North America, despite declining rates of tobacco use, the incidence of head and neck cancers is increasing, likely due to other environmental risk factors such as alcohol use and human papillomavirus infection.[37] Although many patients opt for prophylactic measures to secure their airway, approximately 80,000 patients a year need emergent intervention.[42]

Airway obstruction is the leading cause of death for individuals with head and neck cancers, caused by tumors that narrow the airway to less than 5 mm in diameter.[43] Although malignancies of the head and neck can affect numerous anatomic sites including the oral cavity, nasopharynx, oropharynx, larynx, and hypopharynx, a prospective case study noted that supraglottic lesions were the most likely to interfere with intubation.[37,44,45] Other neoplasms such as lymphomas and anaplastic thyroid cancer can also pose significant challenges during the intubation process.[39]

Anatomic challenges associated with intubation in patients with head and neck cancers are usually secondary to large obstructive tumors that distort airway anatomy. These distortions can be further complicated by common treatments for head and neck cancers, including surgery and radiation therapy. Although a single-center retrospective study failed to show that head and neck radiotherapy is associated with intubation failure, certain advanced airway techniques required to avoid complications (eg, fiberoptic laryngoscopy and bronchoscopy) are often not available in the emergency setting.[40]

Data from the same retrospective study showed that radiotherapy is associated with restrictions in range of motion and trismus.[40] Trismus, caused by radiotherapy-induced tonic contractions and fibrosis to the muscles of mastication, is not receptive to paralytic agents and complicates an already anatomically difficult airway.[40]

Other physiologic challenges associated with airway management in patients with head and neck cancers include lymphadenopathy and bleeding. With approximately 90% of head and neck cancers classified as the squamous cell in origin, primary tumors can metastasize to local lymph nodes, causing significant lymphadenopathy.[46] Neoplasms of the head and neck are also highly vascular and therefore more susceptible to hemorrhage.[47] It is important that clinicians consider the risk of bleeding when manipulating the airway during the intubation process.

Owing to the challenges listed above, emergency clinicians should exercise caution when deciding to intubate patients with head and neck cancers. When available, anesthesia and surgery should be consulted early as failure to secure an endotracheal tube would require surgical intervention.

In addition, ordering or reviewing imaging of the head, neck, and chest before intubation can help localize the obstruction and determine the viability of passing an endotracheal tube. When imaging is not available, the Mallampati score was shown to be a sensitive measurement for difficult tracheal intubation in these patients.[40]

Indications for emergent airway intervention in patients with cancer-related airway obstructions include stridor while at rest. Indicating that greater than 50% of the airway is obstructed, stridor at rest warrants immediate consultation by surgery for possible tracheostomy.[48] Although it is still recommended that these patients be intubated in the operating room, emergency physicians should be ready to act in urgent cases.

Various techniques have been described for intubating patients with malignant airway obstruction; however, most of the literature is based on controlled preoperative cases performed by anesthesiology with little information available on emergency management.

Although widely unavailable in many emergency departments, awake fiberoptic intubation offers several advantages for these patients. Avoiding sedative and paralytic agents preserves intrinsic respiratory function and optimizes oxygenation, whereas fiberoptic capabilities allow clinicians to maneuver around large obstructions. Glycopyrrolate and benzocaine can be used to help decrease secretions and help patients tolerate awake airway manipulation, however short-acting sedatives, such as dopaminergic antipsychotic agents, are recommended when needed.[38] Although ketamine often provides adequate sedation while maintaining spontaneous respirations, it can further complicate an obstructive airway by causing hypersecretions.[38] Other intubation techniques described in the literature but often unavailable in emergency circumstances include awake fibercapnic intubation, cuff inflation, and laser cytoreduction.[39,49]

If intubation fails or the endotracheal tube cannot be secured beyond the level of obstruction, clinicians should be prepared to perform an emergent cricothyrotomy, followed by an emergent tracheostomy in a controlled environment.[39] Laryngeal mask airways are not viable rescue options as the device is usually larger than endotracheal tubes and unlikely to pass the airway obstruction.

Cervical Spine

Traumatic cervical spine considerations

Intubating patients with cervical spine precautions is a common scenario in the emergency department. The utility of spinal immobilization in the general treatment of trauma patients remains unclear and its necessity is equally controversial when it comes to its role in ETI.[50] The data are limited and the studies that exist often take place in the operating room or on cadavers. It is also worth noting that despite the vast amount of debate and precaution taken with these patients, the incidence of neurologic injury secondary to ETI is exceedingly rare, estimated to be 0.03%.[51] However, the concerns about performing ETI on patients with spinal injuries continue to inform guidelines for the procedure.

Patients with confirmed, suspected, or possible traumatic cervical spine injury (CSI) may require ETI for several reasons. Injury to the cervical spine can cause anatomic disruption and local swelling leading to airway compromise.[52] A high CSI can lead to diaphragmatic weakness or paralysis, impairing ventilation and oxygenation. Injury to the spinal cord itself can cause neurogenic shock resulting in altered mental status and inability to maintain airway patency. These injuries also rarely occur in isolation, meaning patients may require intubation for a completely different reason (head trauma, maxillofacial trauma, and so forth), but still must be treated as if they have a possible CSI.[53]

The primary concern with laryngoscopy in patients with possible CSI is the amount of cervical spine movement it may generate, and if that movement can induce or worsen injury to the cord. Paradoxically, concerted efforts are made to prevent spinal movement, thereby making laryngoscopy more difficult.[54]

In isolation, laryngoscopy causes minimal spinal movement in both injured and un-injured patients, although maneuvers to position these patients require significantly more movement.[55] Several studies of laryngoscopy in patients with injured spines reveal that cervical vertebrae typically moved between 1 and 3 mm during laryngos-copy, although many of these patients were immobilized during the procedure either by way of manual in-line immobilization or a cervical spine collar. In examining DL versus VL, they found that VL typically resulted in even less movement of the spine and a better view of the vocal cords, although the time to intubation was increased. In contrast to these reports of minimal movement, one study identified more than 6 mm of narrowing in the spinal canal during flexion and extension of an injured spine, which may have implications on pre-intubation positioning and preoxygenation.[56]

In addition to data showing the minimal movement of the cervical spine during laryn-goscopy, data also fail to consistently show benefits from spinal stabilization. A recent review provides a summary of available, low-quality evidence regarding the impact of spinal stabilization during intubation, and the authors conclude that manual stabiliza-tion of the cervical spine may be ineffective and may hinder intubation.[57]

Despite the minimal amount of spinal movement observed, the unclear benefit of manual immobilization, the hindrance of cervical spine immobilization, and the low incidence of ETI-induced spinal injury, the American College of Surgeons, EAST, and the Western Trauma Association recommend in-line cervical spine stabilization during the intubation of these patients.[58,59]

The ideal method of intubation of patients with confirmed, suspected, or possible CSI is unclear. A survey of anesthesiologists showed that most would prefer to intu-bate these patients with fiberoptic technology,[5] although it seems obvious why this would not be feasible for acutely ill trauma patients in the emergency department. Instead, we are left with recommendations from our trauma colleagues, although at times these feel unclear as well. For example, the EAST makes a Level 1 recommen-dation for standard RSI with DL, but later offers a lower level recommendation that reads, "Video laryngoscopy may offer significant advantages over DL."[54]

Because of continued uncertainty regarding best practices for intubating patients with confirmed or possible cervical spine injuries, physicians should continue to plan ahead for these intubations and reflect on what methods will best facilitate their own success. Emergency departments and trauma surgery departments should collaborate to establish joint policies on airway management in these patients.

Atraumatic cervical spine considerations

Some patients may require consideration of cervical spine manipulation during intuba-tion, even in the absence of traumatic injury. One of these populations is patients with Down syndrome (DS). Although the incidence of intubation-induced CSI in this population is not known, available data and case reports indicate that it is extremely rare.[60] However, there are special considerations when performing laryngoscopy in these patients.

Patients with DS have a higher frequency of various complicated airway features, with particular concern for cervical spine instability.[61] Ligamentous laxity between C1 and C2 (atlantoaxial instability) can be easily disrupted with neck manipulation and may potentially injure the spinal cord. Approximately 20% of these patients can have atlantoaxial instability, although only 1% to 2% may be symptomatic and display neurologic symptoms.[62] This instability can be exacerbated and disrupted by ETI, leaving patients vulnerable to spinal injury.

The anesthesia literature advocates for a neutral position during intubation, with some authors suggesting placement of a "soft collar," whereas some simply remark on maintaining "inline stabilization" during the intubation, in addition to using other adjuncts (securing head to bed, using supports on the side of the head to prevent rotation).[63,64]

The ideal modality to be used during these intubations remains unclear. Data are extremely limited in this group, and it is only recently that patients with DS regularly survive into adulthood. In the emergent intubation of a patient with DS, hyperangulated VL may be the ideal option for reducing cervical spine movement.

Another condition that may impact atlantoaxial stability, as well as other areas of the cervical spine, is rheumatoid arthritis (RA). Like DS, neurologic sequelae from laryngoscopy is considered rare, with one review article from 2011 stating there were no case reports written.[65]

Fiberoptic intubation seems to be the method of choice for anesthesiologists intubating patients with RA.[61,66] This may be an impossibility in the emergency department for several reasons, including resources, training, and the acuity of the patient.

The same precautions taken with patients suffering from DS should be applied to those with RA for similar reasons, and it is likely that hyperangulated VL is a reasonable choice. However, patients with RA may also have dysmorphic anatomy that leads to extremely difficult pre-intubation positioning. The emergency physician should consider how much manipulation and force might be necessary to appropriately position the patient for ETI with conventional intubation techniques. It may be wise to consider flexible endoscopic intubation in patients who are difficult to position, and preparing for a surgical airway if need be.

SUMMARY

The term "anatomically difficult airway" is one that encompasses a vast amount of deformities that the emergency physician may face when intubating a critically ill patient. The specific management of patients with difficult airway features can be guided by the features of the specific deformities, although many recommendations remain based on expert opinions and weak data, often obtained outside the emergency department. Physicians managing these airways should give careful consideration to various airway modalities and choose a technique based on pathology, resources, and experience.

CLINICS CARE POINTS

- When approaching a grossly contaminated airway, consider delayed sequence intubation for nasogastric tube placement, bed-up-head-elevated positioning (BUHE) and the "Suction-Assisted Laryngoscopy for Airway Decontamination" technique.

- Clinicians can refer to the Denver criteria for a list of criteria when considering the intubation of a patient with significant burns.
- Patients suffering from anaphylaxis or angioedema are unlikely to require intubation if only the face and lips are involved.
- For all patients with dynamic airway features, a fiberoptic approach is a reasonable first-line intubation technique—for patients with penetrating neck trauma, rapid sequence intubation may also be reasonable.
- When intubating patients with obesity, put them in the BUHE. This may help laryngoscopy views and prolong the time it takes for them to desaturate.
- Pregnant women have increased metabolic demands and lower functional residual capacity, leading to quicker desaturation times. The BUHE position may be beneficial in this population to stave off desaturation.
- Airway obstruction is the leading cause of death in patients with head and neck cancers. Emergency physicians should consider early consultation of their anesthesia and surgery colleagues when faced with impending airway compromise.
- In patients with cervical spine instability due to injury or disease, fiberoptic intubation is a reasonable approach. However, in the emergent airway, aside from maintaining in-line stabilization, there are minimal data on best the best intubation method. Clinicians should consider their resources, training, and competency levels.

ACKNOWLEDGMENT

Special thanks to Dr. Ananad Swaminathan for his contributions to this article.

DISCLOSURE

The authors have nothing to disclose.

REFERENCES

1. Detsky ME, Jivraj N, Adhikari NK, et al. Will this patient be difficult to intubate? The rational clinical examination systematic review. JAMA 2019;321(5):493–503.
2. Bucher JT, Cooper JS. Bag mask ventilation (Bag Valve Mask, BVM). In: Stat-Pearls. Treasure Island (FL): StatPearls Publishing; 2019. Available at: https://www.ncbi.nlm.nih.gov/books/NBK441924/.
3. Lane S, Saunders D, Schofield A, et al. A prospective, randomised controlled trial comparing the efficacy of pre-oxygenation in the 20° head-up vs supine position. Anaesthesia 2005;60(11):1064–7.
4. Dixon BJ, Dixon JB, Carden JR, et al. Preoxygenation Is More Effective in the 25° Head-up Position Than in the Supine Position in Severely Obese Patients. Anesthesiology 2005;102(6):1110–5 [discussion: 5A].
5. Khandelwal N, Khorsand S, Mitchell SH, et al. Head-Elevated Patient Positioning Decreases Complications of Emergent Tracheal Intubation in the Ward and Intensive Care Unit. Anesth Analg 2016;122(4):1101–7.
6. Stoecklein HH, Kelly C, Kaji AH, et al. Multicenter Comparison of Nonsupine Versus Supine Positioning During Intubation in the Emergency Department: A National Emergency Airway Registry (NEAR) Study. Acad Emerg Med 2019;26(10):1144–51.
7. Suction Assisted Laryngoscopy and Airway Decontamination (SALAD). Available at: https://www.sscor.com/suction-assisted-laryngoscopy-and-airway-decontamination-salad. Accessed November 30, 2019.

8. American Burn Association. Available at: http://ameriburn.org/wp-content/uploads/2019/08/2018-abls-providermanual.pdf. Accessed October 28, 2021.
9. Bittner EA, Shank E, Woodson L, et al. Acute and perioperative care of the burn-injured patient. Anesthesiology 2015;122(2):448–64.
10. Romanowski KS, Palmieri TL, Sen S, et al. More Than One Third of Intubations in Patients Transferred to Burn Centers are Unnecessary: Proposed Guidelines for Appropriate Intubation of the Burn Patient. J Burn Care Res 2016;37(5):e409–14.
11. Dingle LA, Wain RAJ, Bishop S, et al. Intubation in burns patients: a 5-year review of the Manchester regional burns centre experience. Burns 2021;47(3):576–86.
12. Eastman AL, Arnoldo BA, Hunt JL, et al. Pre-burn center management of the burned airway: do we know enough? J Burn Care Res 2010;31(5):701–5.
13. Madnani DD, Steele NP, de Vries E. Factors that predict the need for intubation in patients with smoke inhalation injury. Ear Nose Throat J 2006;85(4):278–80.
14. Badulak JH, Schurr M, Sauaia A, et al. Defining the criteria for intubation of the patient with thermal burns. Burns 2018;44(3):531–8.
15. Orozco-Peláez, Yuliana Aa, b,c d. Airway burn or inhalation injury: should all patients be intubated? Colombian J Anesthesiol 2018;46(2S):26–31.
16. Kameda T, Fujita M. Point-of-care ultrasound detection of tracheal wall thickening caused by smoke inhalation. Crit Ultrasound J 2014;6(1):11.
17. Ishoo E, Shah UK, Grillone GA, et al. Predicting airway risk in angioedema: staging system based on presentation. Otolaryngol Head Neck Surg 1999;121(3):263–8.
18. World Allergy Organization (WAO). Available at: https://www.worldallergyorganizationjournal.org/action/showPdf?pii=S1939-4551%2820%2930375-6. Accessed October 28, 2021.
19. Greenberger PA, Rotskoff BD, Lifschultz B. Fatal anaphylaxis: postmortem findings and associated comorbid diseases. Ann Allergy Asthma Immunol 2007;98(3):252–7.
20. Bishop S, Maguire S. Anaesthesia and intensive care for major burns. Continuing Education Anaesth Crit Care Pain 2012;12(3). https://doi.org/10.1093/bjaceaccp/mks001.
21. Moellman JJ, Bernstein JA, Lindsell C, et al. A consensus parameter for the evaluation and management of angioedema in the emergency department. Acad Emerg Med 2014;21(4):469–84.
22. Sandefur BJ, Liu XW, Kaji AH, et al. Emergency Department Intubations in Patients With Angioedema: A Report from the National Emergency Airway Registry [published online ahead of print, 2021 Aug 31]. J Emerg Med 2021. https://doi.org/10.1016/j.jemermed.2021.07.012. S0736-4679(21)00549-7.
23. Driver BE, Prekker ME, Reardon RF, et al. Success and Complications of the Ketamine-Only Intubation Method in the Emergency Department. J Emerg Med 2021;60(3):265–72.
24. Mayglothling J, Duane TM, Gibbs M, et al. Emergency tracheal intubation immediately following traumatic injury. J Trauma Acute Care Surg 2012;73(5):S333–40.
25. Mandavia DP, Qualls S, Rokos I. Emergency airway management in penetrating neck injury. Ann Emerg Med 2000;35(3):221–5.
26. Nowicki JL, Stew B, Ooi E. Penetrating neck injuries: a guide to evaluation and management. Ann R Coll Surg Engl 2018;100(1):6–11.
27. Dargin J, Medzon R. Emergency department management of the airway in obese adults. Ann Emerg Med 2010;56(2):95–104.
28. Bond A. Obesity and difficult intubation. Anaesth Intensive Care 1993;21(6):828–30.

29. Karkouti K, Rose DK, Wigglesworth D, et al. Predicting difficult intubation: a multi-variable analysis. Can J Anaesth 2000;47(8):730–9.
30. Yildiz TS, Solak M, Toker K. The incidence and risk factors of difficult mask ventilation. Journal of anesthesia 2005;19(1):7–11. https://doi.org/10.1007/s00540-004-0275-z/.
31. Gander S; Frascarolo, P; Suter, M, et al; Positive End-Expiratory Pressure During Induction of General Anesthesia Increases Duration of Nonhypoxic Apnea in Morbidly Obese Patients," Anesth Analg: 2005 Volume 100 - 2 - p 580-584 doi:
32. Dargin JM, Emlet LL, Guyette FX. The effect of body mass index on intubation success rates and complications during emergency airway management. Internal and emergency medicine 2013;8(1):75–82. https://doi.org/10.1007/s11739-012-0874-x.
33. Tsan S, Lim SM, Abidin M, et al. Comparison of Macintosh Laryngoscopy in Bed-up-Head-Elevated Position With GlideScope Laryngoscopy: A Randomized, Controlled, Noninferiority Trial. Anesthesia and analgesia 2020;131(1):210–9. https://doi.org/10.1213/ANE.0000000000004349.
34. Kristensen MS, Teoh WH, Rudolph SS, et al. A randomised cross-over comparison of the transverse and longitudinal techniques for ultrasound-guided identification of the cricothyroid membrane in morbidly obese subjects. Anaesthesia 2016;71(6):675–83.
35. Lapinsky SE. Management of Acute Respiratory Failure in Pregnancy. Semin Respir Crit Care Med 2017;38(2):201–7.
36. Bhatia P, Chhabra S. Physiological and anatomical changes of pregnancy: Implications for anaesthesia. Indian J Anaesth 2018;62(9):651–7.
37. Biro P. Difficult intubation in pregnancy. Curr Opin Anaesthesiol 2011;24(3):249–54.
38. Lee SW, Khaw KS, Ngan Kee WD, et al. Haemodynamic effects from aortocaval compression at different angles of lateral tilt in non-labouring term pregnant women. Br J Anaesth 2012;109(6):950–6.
39. Kodali BS, Chandrasekhar S, Bulich LN, et al. Airway changes during labor and delivery. Anesthesiology 2008;108(3):357–62.
40. Hignett R, Fernando R, McGlennan A, et al. A randomized crossover study to determine the effect of a 30° head-up versus a supine position on the functional residual capacity of term parturients. Anesth Analg 2011;113(5):1098–102.
41. WHO 2014. Available at: https://www.who.int/selection_medicines/committees/expert/20/applications/HeadNeck.pdf. Accessed October 28, 2021.
42. Chen K, Varon J, Wenker OC. Malignant airway obstruction: recognition and management. J Emerg Med 1998;16(1):83–92.
43. Lopez-Gomez J, Gomez-Pedraza A, Granados-Garcia M, et al. Emergency Surgical Treatment of Upper Airway Obstruction in Oncological Patients: Bibliographic Review and Proposal for Management Algorithm. Head Neck Cancer Res 2018;3(1):02.
44. Zheng G, Feng L, Lewis CM. A data review of airway management in patients with oral cavity or oropharyngeal cancer: a single-institution experience. BMC Anesthesiol 2019;19(1):92.
45. Iseli TA, Iseli CE, Golden JB, et al. Outcomes of intubation in difficult airways due to head and neck pathology. Ear Nose Throat J 2012;91(3):E1–5.
46. Sathyanarayan V, Bharani SK. Enlarged lymph nodes in head and neck cancer: Analysis with triplex ultrasonography. Ann Maxillofac Surg 2013;3(1):35–9.
47. Rzewnicki I, Kordecki K, Lukasiewicz A, et al. Palliative embolization of hemorrhages in extensive head and neck tumors. Pol J Radiol 2012;77(4):17–21.

48. Zochios V, Protopapas AD, Valchanov K. Stridor in adult patients presenting from the community: An alarming clinical sign. J Intensive Care Soc 2015;16(3):272–3.
49. Huitink JM, Buitelaar DR, Schutte PFE. Awake fibrecapnic intubation: a novel technique for intubation in head and neck cancer patients with a difficult airway. Anaesthesia 2006;61:449–52.
50. Kwan I, Bunn F, Roberts I. Spinal immobilisation for trauma patients. The Cochrane database of systematic reviews 2001;2001(2):CD002803. https://doi.org/10.1002/14651858.CD002803.
51. Kovacs G, Sowers N. Airway Management in Trauma. Emerg Med Clin North Am 2018;36(1):61–84.
52. Eissa SA, Reed JG, Kortbeek JB, et al. Airway Compromise Secondary to Upper Cervical Spine Injury. J Trauma Inj Infect Crit Care 2009;67(4):692–6.
53. Burney RE, Maio RF, Maynard F, et al. Incidence, characteristics, and outcome of spinal cord injury at trauma centers in North America. Arch Surg 1993;128:596–9.
54. Heath KJ. The effect on laryngoscopy of different cervical spine immobilization techniques. Anaesthesia 1994;49:843–5.
55. Crosby ET, Warltier DC. Airway Management in Adults after Cervical Spine Trauma. Anesthesiology 2006;104:1293–318.
56. Donaldson WF III, Heil BV, Donaldson VP, et al. The Effect of Airway Maneuvers on the Unstable C1-C2 Segment. Spine 1997;22(11):1215–8.
57. Manoach S, Paladino L. Manual In-Line Stabilization for Acute Airway Management of Suspected Cervical Spine Injury: Historical Review and Current Questions. Ann Emerg Med 2007;50(3):236–45.
58. Mayglothling J, Duane TM, Gibbs M, et al. Endotracheal Intubation Following Trauma. J Trauma Acute Care Surg 2012;73(5). Available at: https://www.east.org/education-career-development/practice-management-guidelines/details/endotracheal-intubation-following-trauma.
59. Brown CVR, Inaba K, Shatz DV, et al. Western Trauma Association critical decisions in trauma: airway management in adult trauma patients, Western Trauma Association. 2020. Available at: https://tsaco.bmj.com/content/tsaco/5/1/e000539.full.pdf. Accessed October 28, 2021.
60. Hata T, Todd MM, Weiskopf RB. Cervical Spine Considerations When Anesthetizing Patients with Down Syndrome. Anesthesiology 2005;102:680–5.
61. Hamilton J, Yaneza MM, Clement WA, et al. The prevalence of airway problems in children with Down's syndrome. Int J Pediatr Otorhinolaryngol 2016;81:1–4.
62. Ali FE, Al-Bustan MA, Al-Busairi WA, et al. Cervical spine abnormalities associated with Down syndrome. Int Orthop 2006;30:284–9.
63. Meitzner MC, Skurnowicz JA. Anesthetic Considerations for Patients with Down Syndrome. Am Assoc Nurse Anesthesiol 2005;73(2):103–7.
64. Oliveira M, Machado H. Perioperative management of patients with down syndrome: a review. J Anesth Clin Res 2018;09(04).
65. Samanta R, Shoukrey K, Griffiths R. Rheumatoid arthritis and anaesthesia. Anaesthesia 2011;66(12):1146–59. https://doi.org/10.1111/j.1365-2044.2011.06890.x.
66. Gaszyński T. Airway Management for General Anesthesia in Patients with Rheumatic Diseases – New Possibilities. Reumatologia/Rheumatology 2019;57(2):69–71.

Acute Respiratory Distress Syndrome

Alin Gragossian, DO, MPH[a], Matthew T. Siuba, DO[b],*

KEYWORDS

- ARDS • Respiratory failure • Respiratory support • Mechanical ventilation
- Noninvasive ventilation • High-flow nasal cannula

KEY POINTS

- Acute respiratory distress syndrome (ARDS) occurs in up to 10% of patients with respiratory failure admitted through the emergency department.
- Use of noninvasive respiratory support has proliferated in recent years; clinicians must understand the relative merits and risks of these technologies and know how to recognize signs of failure.
- The cornerstone of ARDS care of the mechanically ventilated patient is low-tidal volume ventilation based on ideal body weight.
- Adjunctive therapies, such as prone positioning and neuromuscular blockade, may have a role in the emergency department management of ARDS depending on patient and department characteristics.
- Recognizing a patient with refractory disease is important to facilitate transfer to an expert center.

BACKGROUND

Acute respiratory distress syndrome (ARDS) is characterized by inflammatory lung injury and carries a global mortality near 40%.[1] It occurs in approximately 6% to 10% of patients with respiratory failure who are admitted through the emergency department.[2,3] Even within the context of the intensive care unit (ICU), the diagnosis is missed in up to half of all patients meeting criteria for the disease.[1] Early recognition is critical to ensure that evidence-based therapies can be implemented without delay.

The most common underlying causes for ARDS, by frequency, commonly encountered in the emergency department include the following: sepsis, pneumonia,

ICMJE Statement: Both A. Gragossian and M.T. Siuba drafted, revised, and approved the final version of this article. No funding was received for this work.
a Department of Critical Care Medicine, The Mount Sinai Hospital, New York, NY, USA;
b Department of Critical Care Medicine, Respiratory Institute, Cleveland Clinic, Cleveland, OH, USA
* Corresponding author. 9500 Euclid Avenue, L2-330, Cleveland, OH 44195.
E-mail address: siubam@ccf.org

aspiration, pancreatitis, blood transfusions, trauma, and burns.[4] Although treating the underlying cause is a cornerstone of ARDS management, there are specific diagnostic and therapeutic considerations that must be pursued as early as possible. Not only are many interventions time sensitive but also the initial care choices in the emergency department often carry over to the ICU upon admission.[5]

DIAGNOSIS
Criteria

ARDS is currently diagnosed using the Berlin definition (**Table 1**).[6] In brief, it is characterized by an acute onset of respiratory illness (within 1 week) with bilateral opacities, which cannot completely be explained by hydrostatic pulmonary edema, with a partial pressure of oxygen to fraction of inspired oxygen ratio ($Pao_2:Fio_2$ ratio) of 300 mm of mercury or less. The current definition requires the application of at least 5 cm of water of positive airway pressure, delivered either via noninvasive positive pressure ventilation (NIV) or via invasive mechanical ventilation (IMV). Given the increase in the use of high-flow nasal cannula (HFNC) over the past decade, it has been proposed to include patients on HFNC in the definition,[7] although currently the Berlin criteria remain the standard (see **Table 1**).

Imaging

Radiograph is usually sufficient for chest imaging to evaluate a patient for ARDS. Although chest computed tomography (CT) is not necessarily required to diagnose ARDS, it may help better characterize the pulmonary parenchyma and possibly identify an underlying cause. Furthermore, contrasted CT scan could identify comorbid pulmonary emboli, which would likely alter therapy. Small series report concurrent pulmonary emboli to be 17% to 39% of the time in patients with COVID-19 ARDS.[8,9]

A more recent development in the diagnosis of ARDS includes the use of point-of-care ultrasound by the bedside clinician using a combination of both lung ultrasound and echocardiography. ARDS can be detected by lung ultrasonography through the recognition of a pulmonary interstitial pattern, which includes the following: B lines with inhomogeneous and gravity-independent distribution, spared areas, pleural line thickening with decreased lung sliding, and subpleural consolidations.[10] Lung ultrasound performs reasonably well in terms of sensitivity and specificity (82.7% to 92.3% and 90.2% to 98.6%, respectively) in ARDS when compared with chest CT.[11] It also provides the ability for real-time monitoring of changes to vent settings,

Table 1 The Berlin definition of acute respiratory distress syndrome	
Timing	Within 1 wk of known insult, or new or worsening symptoms
Chest imaging	Bilateral opacities not fully explained by pleural effusions, lobar collapse, or nodules
Origin of edema	Respiratory failure not fully explained by cardiac failure or fluid overload. Objective assessment is required
Oxygenation (measured on at least 5 cm H_2O PEEP or CPAP)	
Mild	200 mm Hg < $Pao_2:Fio_2$ ≤ 300 mm Hg
Moderate	100 mm Hg < $Pao_2:Fio_2$ ≤ 200 mm Hg
Severe	100 mm Hg ≤ $Pao_2:Fio_2$

Abbreviation: CPAP, continuous positive airway pressure.

such as positive end expiratory pressure (PEEP) titration,[12–14] although this is not commonly used. Importantly, lung ultrasound would not be able to differentiate between well-aerated lung and overdistended lung, as both would result in an A-line pattern.

Focused cardiac ultrasound can also be used to establish the diagnosis (ie, rule out cardiogenic pulmonary edema), as well as monitor the effect of ARDS on the right ventricle. Right ventricular dysfunction can be seen in 22% to 27% of patients with ARDS.[15,16] Right heart failure owing to increased pulmonary vascular resistance (acute cor pulmonale) is characterized by right-ventricle dilatation and septal dyskinesia on echocardiography.[17] Moreover, a coexisting patent foramen ovale with shunt can occur in nearly 20% of patients with ARDS and may be responsible for a higher rate of refractory hypoxemia and an increased number of ventilator-dependent days.[18] Discovering a shunt in the patient with ARDS may also alter therapy, whereby the pulmonary vascular resistance should be lowered as much as possible to decrease shunt fraction.

MANAGEMENT

Treatment of the underlying condition that led to ARDS is the primary management consideration. The remainder of care is largely supportive and centers on the careful application of respiratory assistance.

Noninvasive Respiratory Support

High-flow nasal cannula

HFNC has gained traction over the past decade, in large part to a multicenter trial showing decreased mortality compared with NIV and standard oxygen therapy in patients with acute hypoxemic respiratory failure[19] as well as improved patient comfort compared with NIV and IMV. A clinical practice guideline has strongly endorsed HFNC over standard oxygen therapy for hypoxemic respiratory failure, as its use has been associated with reduction in intubation rates and escalation of respiratory support.[20] Use can be considered in patients with ARDS if airway protective reflexes are intact and the patient is hemodynamically stable. Benefits include decreased respiratory effort, in part because of washout of anatomic dead space. Flow rate (in liters per minute) can be titrated to patient comfort, and administered Fio_2 (up to 1.0) can be adjusted based on oxygen saturation targets. Close monitoring of patients on HFNC is necessary, so patients may require admission to ICUs or intermediate care units depending on local resources. A metric used to predict HFNC failure is the ROX index ([oxygen saturation/Fio_2]/respiratory rate).[21] A value of 4.88 or above from 2 to 12 hours after application of HFNC was associated with a lower risk of intubation. Values associated with HFNC failure at different time points are reported in **Table 2**. It is important to note that this scoring system does not take work of breathing into account, and clinical assessment is needed to determine whether ongoing HFNC therapy is appropriate.

Noninvasive ventilation

Noninvasive ventilation is frequently used in patients with ARDS, although its use remains controversial. The potential benefits include avoidance of ventilator-associated events and need for deep sedation, which often come with IMV. In addition, appropriately titrated end expiratory pressure could decrease injury related to vigorous spontaneous breathing.[22] Potential harms include delayed (necessary) intubation, inability to control tidal volumes and monitor airway pressures, and inconsistent mask seal, which could lead to cyclic recruitment-derecruitment of lung units causing

Table 2 ROX score to predict high-flow nasal cannula failure	
Time Point, h	**Likely Failure Value**
2	2.85
6	3.47
12	3.85

ROX score is calculated as the ratio of oxygen saturation/fraction of inspired oxygen over respiratory rate. A patient with oxygen saturation of 90% on fraction of inspired oxygen of 0.70 with a respiratory rate of 24 would have the value (90/0.7)/24 = 5.36.

atelectrauma. A small randomized trial in patients with moderate to severe ARDS using a full-helmet interface showed reduction in rate of intubation as well as mortality when compared with standard facemask NIV.[23] A study in patients with COVID-19 ARDS using helmet interface (compared with HFNC) did not show a mortality benefit, but did demonstrate a reduction in intubation rate as well as ventilator days.[24] Patients in the helmet NIV group frequently required sedation to facilitate comfort. Helmet NIV must be used with a traditional ventilator, as it requires a dual limb circuit (inspiratory and expiratory limbs), and the settings must be adjusted carefully to avoid carbon dioxide rebreathing. Helmet NIV is not routinely available in most North American hospitals, requires familiarity with the technology, and would benefit from further study in pragmatic trials before widespread use.

Most patients receive NIV via facemask interface, with widespread use owing to its strong evidence base for hypercapnic respiratory failure and cardiogenic pulmonary edema. The data on its role in ARDS are conflicting. The RECOVERY-RS trial in patients with COVID ARDS demonstrated a decreased intubation rate, but no mortality benefit, in patients treated with NIV (continuous positive airway pressure, specifically) compared with standard oxygen therapy; the same benefit was not observed when comparing HFNC with standard oxygen therapy.[25] A propensity-matched analysis of the LUNG-SAFE study demonstrated an increased risk of mortality of patients with moderate to severe ARDS who received NIV compared with those who received IMV only.[26] High-quality, prospective randomized trials are needed to better define the role of NIV in ARDS.

Safety monitoring in NIV is essential, and the authors advocate for these patients to be admitted to ICUs when possible. Tidal volume monitoring plays an important role. Patients with moderate to severe hypoxemia and tidal volumes greater than 9.5 mL/kg of ideal body weight (IBW) despite attempts to lower the tidal volume by changing settings are expected to fail NIV (82% sensitivity, 87% specificity).[27] The HACOR score (Heart rate, Acidosis, Consciousness, Oxygenation, Respiratory rate) predicts failure of NIV in patients with hypoxemic respiratory failure.[28] A summary of the score and its value at different timepoints can be found at this referenced summary[29]; the score itself is listed in **Table 3**. Score at 1 hour may also help differentiate patients who may be less likely to die if intubated early (within 12 hours of NIV initiation).[28] HACOR scores will tend to improve in patients with NIV success and remain unchanged in patients with NIV failure. The presence of other organ failures may also predict NIV failure.[30] In summary, if a patient with ARDS placed on NIV does not markedly improve, ongoing use in the individual should be reconsidered.

Awake prone positioning

Awake prone positioning became popular during the early portion of the COVID-19 pandemic, despite a lack of meaningful outcome data at that time. Subsequently, a

Table 3
HACOR score to predict noninvasive ventilation failure

Variables	Category	Assigned Points
Heart rate (beats/min)	≤120	0
	>121	1
pH	≥7.35	0
	7.30–7.34	2
	7.25–7.29	3
	<7.25	4
Glascow Coma Scale	15	0
	13–14	2
	11–12	5
	≤10	10
Pao$_2$:Fio$_2$ ratio	≥201	0
	176–200	2
	151–175	3
	126–150	4
	101–125	5
	≤100	6
Respiratory rate (breaths/min)	≤30	0
	31–35	1
	36–40	2
	41–45	3
	≥46	4

multinational randomized "meta-trial" of 1121 patients compared HFNC and awake prone positioning with HFNC alone.[31] There was a 6% absolute reduction in treatment failure (defined as intubation or death) in the prone position group, with no signal of harm detected. Patients who were able to prone for more than 8 hours per day had a lower rate of treatment failure compared with those who were in the prone position for less than 8 hours as well. Although prone, patients had improvement in ROX score as well as its components (SpO$_2$:Fio$_2$ ratio and respiratory rate). This treatment is easy to implement and could be instituted while still in the emergency department, assuming the patient is an otherwise suitable candidate for HFNC and can self-prone without difficulty or excess discomfort. Less is known about the combination of NIV and awake prone positioning.

Invasive mechanical ventilation management

Fig. 1 provides a comprehensive management algorithm. The supporting information for this algorithm is described in the following sections.

Safety parameters

Limiting harm from mechanical ventilation is the highest-priority action. Details on tidal volume and PEEP selection will be detailed subsequently. In general, oxygenation goals include partial pressure of arterial oxygen (Pao$_2$) target between 55 and 80 mm Hg or pulse oximetry (SpO$_2$) values from 88% to 95%. Permissive hypercapnia is generally well tolerated and may actually be protective.[32] Various lower limits for pH have been described (anywhere from 7.15 to 7.25), although no specific threshold is supported by strong evidence. Plateau pressure, a surrogate for compliance of the respiratory system, should be kept less than 30 cm H$_2$O.[33] This value can be obtained by initiating a brief (0.5 second) inspiratory pause on the ventilator, during passive

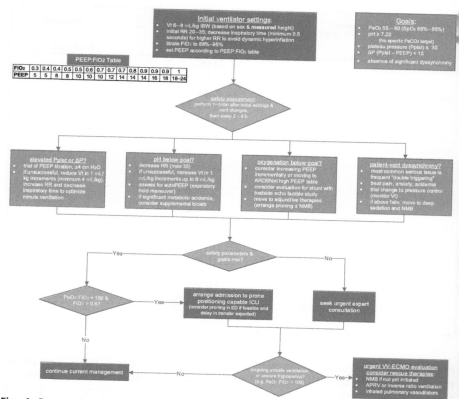

Fig. 1. Proposed management algorithm for ARDS in the emergency department. ΔP, driving pressure; ED, emergency department; max, maximum; Paco₂, partial pressure of arterial carbon dioxide; Pplat, plateau pressure; RR, respiratory rate; Vt, tidal volume.

ventilation. Observational data also suggest decreased mortality with the driving pressure (the difference between plateau pressure and PEEP) kept lower than 13 to 15 cm H$_2$O.[34–36] Plateau pressure should be rechecked periodically and after each ventilator adjustment; changes to plateau and driving pressures can be observed in as short as 1 to 5 minutes after adjustments are made,[37] although longer time periods are required to see improvements from slow recruitment. More information on these targets and how to reach them is included in **Fig. 1**.

Low-tidal-volume ventilation

Despite more than 2 decades of knowledge that lower tidal volumes are associated with lower mortality,[33] implementation of low-tidal volume ventilation (LTVV) is inconsistent,[1] even in expert centers and with higher severity of disease.[38] Several studies have demonstrated that protocolized care in ARDS is associated with better adherence to LTVV, as well as improved outcomes.[39,40] In fact, similar findings have been demonstrated for protocol-driven ventilator management in the emergency department. LOV-ED, a before-after implementation study, showed a 48% increase in lung-protective ventilation after protocol implementation.[5] Importantly, this protocol also improved adherence to lung protective ventilation of the same patients in the ICU, suggesting a "carry-over" effect. Prompt initiation of LTVV is important, as observational data suggest even early application of higher tidal volumes is associated with higher mortality.[41] It must be emphasized that tidal volume targets should be set based on ideal rather than actual body weight, as patients with obesity are more likely to receive higher tidal volumes.[42] For patients with ARDS, the goal tidal volume range falls between 4 and 8 mL/kg of IBW (starting at 6 mL/kg for most patients).[43]

Positive end expiratory pressure titration
The goal of PEEP titration is to achieve alveolar recruitment without overdistention, thereby homogenizing the alveoli as much as possible. No approach to the titration of PEEP has proven superior to any other in terms of patient-centered outcomes.[44,45] Patients with more severe hypoxemia may have lower mortalities when a higher PEEP strategy is used.[46] In practice, PEEP may be set lower than appropriate, as even patients with severe hypoxemia receive only 10 cm H_2O PEEP on average.[1] Some clinicians may be hesitant to increase PEEP if hemodynamic instability is present, although it is reasonable to still perform a brief trial of PEEP increase to see if it is tolerable and safe by hemodynamics and plateau pressures. Often, changes in oxygenation are used to assess if PEEP titration was helpful, although a "positive" response may be better reflected by a decrease in driving pressure.[34,47] More data are needed to assess strategies of PEEP titration. In general it is reasonable to use the ARDSnet low PEEP table as a starting point (see **Fig. 1**), but to consider the high PEEP table if hypoxemia is more severe.[48] It is essential to monitor plateau and driving pressures, as well as hemodynamics, while titrating PEEP.

Prone position ventilation
The physiologic benefits of prone positioning have been discussed in detail elsewhere,[49] but can be summarized briefly as improving dorsal lung recruitment, overall ventilation/perfusion matching, and homogenizing stress and strain throughout the lung. There may also be hemodynamic benefits as well, because prone positioning tends to offload the right ventricle through a combination of mechanisms.[50] Prone positioning is consistently associated with improved mortality in patients with moderate to severe ARDS,[51,52] especially when paired with LTVV.[53] The largest trial showing mortality benefit, PROSEVA, enrolled patients with moderate to severe ARDS after 12 to 24 hours of optimized mechanical ventilation,[52] which calls into question whether this strategy is needed in patients while still in the emergency department. It may become necessary if long delays in transfer to the ICU or another facility are anticipated, although familiarity with the process is important, as the mortality reduction in PROSEVA was approximately 16%. A process for performing prone positioning in the emergency department has been described elsewhere.[54]

Neuromuscular blockade
The use of neuromuscular blockade (NMB) in patients with moderate to severe ARDS is associated with improved oxygenation, decreased ventilator-associated lung injury, and improved mortality at 28 days, without increasing the incidence of neuromuscular weakness.[55] The most recent multicenter trial of NMB in ARDS (ROSE, data from which are included in Ref.[55]), did not demonstrate a mortality benefit compared with a control group, which only used light sedation, so routine use of NMB has been called into question. NMB use does require deep sedation, which is associated with increased mortality even after accounting for severity of illness, so this strategy must be used cautiously.[56] Optimal usage would likely be in a patient with moderate to severe ARDS who is also having significant ventilator dyssynchrony not amenable to ventilator adjustments. Bolus and/or infusions of NMB agents should be used for the shortest duration possible. In the emergency department, it may be more practical

to use intermittent boluses depending on length of stay. It is also important to note that depth of sedation does not correlate with respiratory drive, so deep sedation without NMB may not be a viable strategy to mitigate dyssynchrony.[57]

Fluid management

A conservative (compared with liberal) fluid strategy in patients with ARDS is associated with fewer days of mechanical ventilation.[58] Patients with ARDS may present with clinical signs of hypoperfusion as well as frank shock. Despite this fact, clinicians should exercise caution with fluid administration, ideally doing so in a targeted fashion (ie, with formal preload responsiveness assessment), if at all.

Corticosteroids

The use of corticosteroids in ARDS remains controversial, owing to decades of conflicting data. Their use has increased after positive clinical trial results for dexamethasone in patients with COVID-19 pneumonia, demonstrating decreased days of mechanical ventilation as well as mortality,[59] as well as a subsequent meta-analysis with compatible results.[60] Similar findings were seen in patients with moderate to severe ARDS, prepandemic, treated with dexamethasone 20 mg for 5 days followed by 10 mg for 5 days, in an open-label, multicenter trial.[61] A meta-analysis that included the aforementioned trial also concluded corticosteroids are associated with decreased mortality and days of mechanical ventilation, without increasing risk of hospital-acquired infections.[62] The decision to initiate corticosteroids (and at what dose) will likely depend on local/institutional factors, and multidisciplinary collaboration is encouraged. It is reasonable to consider steroids earlier in patients with higher severity of illness.

Inhaled pulmonary vasodilators

Inhaled pulmonary vasodilators have been used in ARDS with the intent of reversing hypoxemic vasoconstriction in ventilated lung units. This effect could also lead to decreased pulmonary vascular resistance, and therefore, right ventricular afterload. Unfortunately, these medications have not been shown to have any patient-centered outcome benefit in trials or high-quality observational studies. Nitric oxide may improve oxygenation without any benefit on mortality and potentially increases the risk of acute kidney injury.[63] In addition, nitric oxide is very expensive in the United States. Inhaled prostaglandins, such as epoprostenol, similarly have been shown to improve oxygenation and lower pulmonary artery pressures, without mortality benefit.[64] As such, these medications should be used sparingly (if at all) and could be considered in the following situations: (1) rescue of refractory hypoxemia, (2) coexistent right ventricular dysfunction, and/or (3) coexistent intracardiac shunt.

Airway pressure release ventilation

Airway pressure release ventilation (APRV) is an alternative mode of ventilation that leverages inverse ratio ventilation (inspiratory time greater than expiratory time) and allows spontaneous breathing. Trial data on APRV are sparse, and its use is most supported by a single-center study that demonstrated improved compliance, oxygenation, decreased days of mechanical ventilation, and sedation.[65] The use of APRV cannot be routinely recommended over conventional modes, but could be considered in centers with sufficient expertise to manage the mode, as well as in cases of refractory hypoxemia, especially if the patient is not a candidate for extracorporeal life support.

Extracorporeal life support

Extracorporeal carbon dioxide removal ($ECCO_2R$) is a low-flow form of venovenous support that has been studied in ARDS. An advantage over venovenous extracorporeal membrane oxygenation (VV-ECMO) is the smaller cannula size (15.5 French, slightly larger than a hemodialysis catheter), although it does not provide any oxygenation support. The most recent trial compared usual care with a strategy of using $ECCO_2R$ to achieve ultraprotective tidal volumes (as low as 3 mL/kg IBW). No mortality benefit was seen, and patients in the intervention group required more sedation and NMB and had longer duration of mechanical ventilation.[66] Currently, the use of $ECCO_2R$ is not approved by the Food and Drug Administration and can only be used in the context of a clinical trial or under Emergency Use Authorization.

VV-ECMO has been studied in 2 large multicenter trials, CESAR[67] and EOLIA,[68] with somewhat conflicting results. However, an individual patient data meta-analysis of the 2 trials concluded that VV-ECMO reduces 90-day mortality in patients with severe ARDS (relative risk, 0.75; 95% confidence interval, 0.60–0.94).[69] Notably, the median $Pao_2:Fio_2$ of patients at enrollment in both treatment and control groups was just under 80. VV-ECMO carries significant cost, is invasive, and is associated with increased risk of morbidity owing to cannulation and anticoagulation. Both trials were done in expert centers, an important consideration with evaluating external validity.

APPROACH TO REFRACTORY HYPOXEMIA

No standard definition for refractory hypoxemia exists; some studies have used a $Pao_2:Fio_2$ ratio of less than 60, whereas Fio_2 is set at 1.0.[70] Furthermore, refractory ARDS may be better captured by inclusion of other factors, such as severe respiratory acidemia, unsafe airway pressures (plateau and driving pressure), and right ventricular dysfunction, rather than solely by hypoxemia.

Most concerning is the poor utilization of evidence-based therapies in patients with moderate to severe ARDS. A recent multicenter observational study demonstrated that less than one-third of patients received lung protective ventilation (defined as tidal volume ≤ 6.5 mL/kg IBW and plateau pressure <30 cm H_2O).[38] PEEP is usually lower than recommended targets in these patients as well. Interventions with low quality of evidence, such as inhaled pulmonary vasodilators, are more frequently implemented than prone positioning.[38,70]

The primary considerations for treating a patient with refractory/severe ARDS is sequential implementation of evidence-based therapies, as in **Fig. 1**. Patients who are referred to expert centers may have improved outcomes,[67] so early consultation is recommended. After optimization of tidal volume and PEEP, early prone positioning and NMB should be initiated. If these interventions do not achieve safe airway pressure and gas exchange parameters, consultation with a VV-ECMO center is advised. If the patient is deemed not a candidate for VV-ECMO, alternative modes of ventilation, such as APRV, can be considered, as well as inhaled pulmonary vasodilators.

SUMMARY

ARDS occurs commonly in patients with respiratory failure in the emergency department. Lung protective ventilation strategies as well as early prone position ventilation have the largest impact on mortality. Protocolized care for ARDS, in the emergency department or ICU, is associated with increased adherence to lung protective ventilation and improved outcomes. Other interventions, such as NMB and VV-ECMO, can be considered in a sequential fashion if airway pressure and gas exchange targets cannot be achieved. In challenging or refractory cases, early expert consultation is advised.

CLINICS CARE POINTS

- Evidence based management of ARDS for an intubated patient relies on accurate administration of low tidal volume ventilation based on ideal body weight.
- There is no "best" strategy for PEEP titration. The PEEP:FiO2 table is a reasonable place to start.

DISCLOSURE

The authors have no financial conflicts of interest.

REFERENCES

1. Bellani G, Laffey JG, Pham T, et al. Epidemiology, Patterns of care, and mortality for patients with acute respiratory distress syndrome in intensive care units in 50 countries. JAMA 2016;315(8):788.
2. Fuller BM, Mohr NM, Dettmer M, et al. Mechanical ventilation and acute lung injury in emergency department patients with severe sepsis and septic shock: an observational study. Acad Emerg Med Off J Soc Acad Emerg Med 2013; 20(7):659–69.
3. Fuller BM, Mohr NM, Miller CN, et al. Mechanical Ventilation and ARDS in the ED: A multicenter, observational, prospective, cross-sectional study. Chest 2015; 148(2):365–74.
4. Rubenfeld GD, Caldwell E, Peabody E, et al. Incidence and outcomes of acute lung injury. N Engl J Med 2005;353(16):1685–93.
5. Fuller BM, Ferguson IT, Mohr NM, et al. Lung-protective ventilation initiated in the emergency department (LOV-ED): a quasi-experimental, before-after trial. Ann Emerg Med 2017;70(3):406–18, e4.
6. ARDS Definition Task Force, Ranieri VM, Rubenfeld GD, et al. Acute respiratory distress syndrome. JAMA 2012;307(23):2526–33.
7. Matthay MA, Thompson BT, Ware LB. The Berlin definition of acute respiratory distress syndrome: should patients receiving high-flow nasal oxygen be included? Lancet Respir Med 2021;9(8):933–6.
8. Soumagne T, Winiszewski H, Besch G, et al. Pulmonary embolism among critically ill patients with ARDS due to COVID-19. Respir Med Res 2020;78:100789.
9. Contou D, Pajot O, Cally R, et al. Pulmonary embolism or thrombosis in ARDS COVID-19 patients: a French monocenter retrospective study. PLoS ONE 2020; 15(8):e0238413.
10. Copetti R, Soldati G, Copetti P. Chest sonography: a useful tool to differentiate acute cardiogenic pulmonary edema from acute respiratory distress syndrome. Cardiovasc Ultrasound 2008;6(1):16.
11. Chiumello D, Umbrello M, Sferrazza Papa GF, et al. Global and regional diagnostic accuracy of lung ultrasound compared to CT in patients with acute respiratory distress syndrome. Crit Care Med 2019;47(11):1599–606.
12. Chiumello D, Cressoni M, Carlesso E, et al. Bedside selection of positive end-expiratory pressure in mild, moderate, and severe acute respiratory distress syndrome. Crit Care Med 2014;42(2):252–64.
13. Algieri I, Mongodi S, Chiumello D, et al. CT scan and ultrasound comparative assessment of PEEP-induced lung aeration changes in ARDS. Crit Care 2014; 18(1):P285.

14. Bouhemad B, Brisson H, Le-Guen M, et al. Bedside ultrasound assessment of positive end-expiratory pressure-induced lung recruitment. Am J Respir Crit Care Med 2011;183(3):341–7.
15. Osman D, Monnet X, Castelain V, et al. Incidence and prognostic value of right ventricular failure in acute respiratory distress syndrome. Intensive Care Med 2009;35(1):69–76.
16. Mekontso Dessap A, Boissier F, Charron C, et al. Acute cor pulmonale during protective ventilation for acute respiratory distress syndrome: prevalence, predictors, and clinical impact. Intensive Care Med 2016;42(5):862–70. Available at: https://dx.doi.org.ccmain.ohionet.org/10.1007/s00134-015-4141-2.
17. Boissier F, Katsahian S, Razazi K, et al. Prevalence and prognosis of cor pulmonale during protective ventilation for acute respiratory distress syndrome. Intensive Care Med 2013;39(10):1725–33.
18. Mekontso Dessap A, Boissier F, Leon R, et al. Prevalence and prognosis of shunting across patent foramen ovale during acute respiratory distress syndrome. Crit Care Med 2010;38(9):1786–92.
19. Frat JP, Thille AW, Mercat A, et al. High-flow oxygen through nasal cannula in acute hypoxemic respiratory failure. N Engl J Med 2015;372(23):2185–96.
20. Rochwerg B, Einav S, Chaudhuri D, et al. The role for high flow nasal cannula as a respiratory support strategy in adults: a clinical practice guideline. Intensive Care Med 2020;46(12):2226–37.
21. Roca O, Caralt B, Messika J, et al. An index combining respiratory rate and oxygenation to predict outcome of nasal high-flow therapy. Am J Respir Crit Care Med 2019;199(11):1368–76.
22. Morais CCA, Koyama Y, Yoshida T, et al. High positive end-expiratory pressure renders spontaneous effort noninjurious. Am J Respir Crit Care Med 2018; 197(10):1285–96.
23. Patel BK, Wolfe KS, Pohlman AS, et al. Effect of noninvasive ventilation delivered by helmet vs face mask on the rate of endotracheal intubation in patients with acute respiratory distress syndrome. JAMA 2016;315(22):2435.
24. Effect of helmet noninvasive ventilation vs high-flow nasal oxygen on days free of respiratory support in patients with COVID-19 and moderate to severe hypoxemic respiratory failure: the HENIVOT randomized clinical trial | critical care medicine | JAMA | JAMA Network. Available at: https://jamanetwork.com/journals/jama/fullarticle/2778088. Accessed November 6, 2021.
25. An adaptive randomized controlled trial of non-invasive respiratory strategies in acute respiratory failure patients with COVID-19 | medRxiv. Available at: https://www.medrxiv.org/content/10.1101/2021.08.02.21261379v1.full.   Accessed November 6, 2021.
26. Bellani G, Laffey JG, Pham T, et al. Noninvasive ventilation of patients with acute respiratory distress syndrome. Insights from the LUNG SAFE study. Am J Respir Crit Care Med 2017;195(1):67–77.
27. Carteaux G, Millán-Guilarte T, De Prost N, et al. Failure of noninvasive ventilation for de novo acute hypoxemic respiratory failure: role of tidal volume. Crit Care Med 2016;44(2):282–90.
28. Duan J, Han X, Bai L, et al. Assessment of heart rate, acidosis, consciousness, oxygenation, and respiratory rate to predict noninvasive ventilation failure in hypoxemic patients. Intensive Care Med 2017;43(2).
29. Predicting NIV failure in hypoxemic patients: the HACOR score. ESICM Published; 2017. Available at: https://www.esicm.org/article-review-icm-hacor-score-feb-2017/. Accessed November 6, 2021.

30. Rodríguez A, Ferri C, Martin-Loeches I, et al. Risk factors for noninvasive ventilation failure in critically III subjects with confirmed influenza infection. Respir Care 2017;62(10):1307–15.

31. Ehrmann S, Li J, Ibarra-Estrada M, et al. Awake prone positioning for COVID-19 acute hypoxaemic respiratory failure: a randomised, controlled, multinational, open-label meta-trial. Lancet Respir Med 2021;0(0). https://doi.org/10.1016/S2213-2600(21)00356-8.

32. O'Croinin D, Ni Chonghaile M, Higgins B, et al. Bench-to-bedside review: permissive hypercapnia. Crit Care 2005;9(1):51–9.

33. Acute Respiratory Distress Syndrome Network, Brower RG, Matthay MA, et al. Ventilation with lower tidal volumes as compared with traditional tidal volumes for acute lung injury and the acute respiratory distress syndrome. N Engl J Med 2000;342(18):1301–8.

34. Amato MBP, Meade MO, Slutsky AS, et al. Driving pressure and survival in the acute respiratory distress syndrome. N Engl J Med 2015;372(8):747–55.

35. Guérin C, Papazian L, Reignier J, et al. Effect of driving pressure on mortality in ARDS patients during lung protective mechanical ventilation in two randomized controlled trials. Crit Care 2016;20(1):384.

36. Goligher EC, Costa ELV, Yarnell CJ, et al. Effect of lowering tidal volume on mortality in ARDS varies with respiratory system elastance. Am J Respir Crit Care Med 2021;13. https://doi.org/10.1164/rccm.202009-3536OC.

37. Sahetya SK, Hager DN, Stephens RS, et al. PEEP titration to minimize driving pressure in subjects with ARDS: a prospective physiological study. Respir Care 2020;65(5):583–9. https://doi.org/10.4187/respcare.07102.

38. Qadir N, Bartz RR, Cooter ML, et al. Variation in early management practices in moderate-to-severe ARDS in the United States: the severe ARDS: generating evidence study. Chest 2021;160(4):1304–15.

39. Duggal A, Panitchote A, Siuba M, et al. Implementation of Protocolized Care in ARDS Improves Outcomes. Respir Care 2020. https://doi.org/10.4187/respcare.07999. Published online.

40. Gallo de Moraes A, Holets SR, Tescher AN, et al. The Clinical effect of an early, protocolized approach to mechanical ventilation for severe and refractory hypoxemia. Respir Care 2020;65(4):413–9.

41. Needham DM, Yang T, Dinglas VD, et al. Timing of low tidal volume ventilation and intensive care unit mortality in acute respiratory distress syndrome. a prospective cohort study. Am J Respir Crit Care Med 2015;191(2):177–85.

42. Kalra SS, Siuba M, Panitchote A, et al. Higher class of obesity is associated with delivery of higher tidal volumes in subjects with ARDS. Respir Care 2020;65(10):1519–26.

43. NHLBI ARDS Network | Tools. Available at: http://ardsnet.org/tools.shtml. Accessed November 7, 2021.

44. Yi H, Li X, Mao Z, et al. Higher PEEP versus lower PEEP strategies for patients in ICU without acute respiratory distress syndrome: a systematic review and meta-analysis. J Crit Care 2022;67:72–8.

45. Walkey AJ, Del Sorbo L, Hodgson CL, et al. Higher PEEP versus lower PEEP strategies for patients with acute respiratory distress syndrome. a systematic review and meta-analysis. Ann Am Thorac Soc 2017;14(Supplement_4):S297–303.

46. Briel M, Meade M, Mercat A, et al. Higher vs lower positive end-expiratory pressure in patients with acute lung injury and acute respiratory distress syndrome. JAMA 2010;303(9):865.

47. Yehya N, Hodgson CL, Amato MBP, et al. Response to ventilator adjustments for predicting acute respiratory distress syndrome mortality. driving pressure versus oxygenation. Ann Am Thorac Soc 2020;18(5):857–64.
48. Fan E, Del Sorbo L, Goligher EC, et al. An official American Thoracic Society/European Society of Intensive Care Medicine/Society of Critical Care Medicine clinical practice guideline: mechanical ventilation in adult patients with acute respiratory distress syndrome. Am J Respir Crit Care Med 2017;195(9):1253–63.
49. Gattinoni L, Taccone P, Carlesso E, et al. Prone position in acute respiratory distress syndrome. rationale, indications, and limits. Am J Respir Crit Care Med 2013;188(11):1286–93.
50. Paternot A, Repessé X, Vieillard-Baron A. Rationale and description of right ventricle-protective ventilation in ARDS. Respir Care 2016;61(10):1391–6.
51. Munshi L, Del Sorbo L, Adhikari NKJ, et al. Prone position for acute respiratory distress syndrome. A systematic review and meta-analysis. Ann Am Thorac Soc 2017;14(Supplement_4):S280–8.
52. Guérin C, Reignier J, Richard JC, et al. Prone positioning in severe acute respiratory distress syndrome. N Engl J Med 2013;368(23):2159–68.
53. Sud S, Friedrich JO, Adhikari NK, et al. Comparative effectiveness of protective ventilation strategies for moderate and severe ARDS: network meta-analysis. Am J Respir Crit Care Med 2021;6. https://doi.org/10.1164/rccm.202008-3039OC.
54. McGurk K, Riveros T, Johnson N, et al. A primer on proning in the emergency department. J Am Coll Emerg Physicians Open 2020;1(6):1703–8.
55. Torbic H, Krishnan S, Harnegie MP, et al. Neuromuscular blocking agents for ARDS: a systematic review and meta-analysis. Respir Care 2021;66(1):120–8.
56. Stephens RJ, Dettmer MR, Roberts BW, et al. Practice patterns and outcomes associated with early sedation depth in mechanically ventilated patients: a systematic review and meta-analysis. Crit Care Med 2018;46(3):471–9.
57. Dzierba AL, Khalil AM, Derry KL, et al. Discordance between respiratory drive and sedation depth in critically Ill patients receiving mechanical ventilation. Crit Care Med 2021;27. https://doi.org/10.1097/CCM.0000000000005113.
58. National Heart, Lung, and Blood Institute Acute Respiratory Distress Syndrome (ARDS) Clinical Trials Network, Wiedemann HP, Wheeler AP, et al. Comparison of two fluid-management strategies in acute lung injury. N Engl J Med 2006;354(24):2564–75.
59. Dexamethasone in hospitalized patients with Covid-19. N Engl J Med 2021;384(8):693–704.
60. The WHO rapid evidence appraisal for COVID-19 therapies (REACT) working group. Association between administration of systemic corticosteroids and mortality among critically ill patients with COVID-19: A meta-analysis. JAMA 2020;324(13):1330–41.
61. Villar J, Ferrando C, Martínez D, et al. Dexamethasone treatment for the acute respiratory distress syndrome: a multicentre, randomised controlled trial. Lancet Respir Med 2020;8(3):267–76.
62. Zayed Y, Barbarawi M, Ismail E, et al. Use of glucocorticoids in patients with acute respiratory distress syndrome: a meta-analysis and trial sequential analysis. J Intensive Care 2020;8(1):43.
63. Karam O, Gebistorf F, Wetterslev J, et al. The effect of inhaled nitric oxide in acute respiratory distress syndrome in children and adults: a Cochrane Systematic Review with trial sequential analysis. Anaesthesia 2017;72(1):106–17.

64. Fuller BM, Mohr NM, Skrupky L, et al. The use of inhaled prostaglandins in patients with ARDS. Chest 2015;147(6):1510–22.
65. Zhou Y, Jin X, Lv Y, et al. Early application of airway pressure release ventilation may reduce the duration of mechanical ventilation in acute respiratory distress syndrome. Intensive Care Med 2017;43(11):1648–59.
66. McNamee JJ, Gillies MA, Barrett NA, et al. Effect of lower tidal volume ventilation facilitated by extracorporeal carbon dioxide removal vs standard care ventilation on 90-day mortality in patients with acute hypoxemic respiratory failure: the rest randomized clinical trial. JAMA 2021;326(11):1013–23.
67. Peek GJ, Mugford M, Tiruvoipati R, et al. Efficacy and economic assessment of conventional ventilatory support versus extracorporeal membrane oxygenation for severe adult respiratory failure (CESAR): a multicentre randomised controlled trial. Lancet 2009;374(9698):1351–63.
68. Combes A, Hajage D, Capellier G, et al. Extracorporeal membrane oxygenation for severe acute respiratory distress syndrome. N Engl J Med 2018;378(21):1965–75.
69. Combes A, Peek GJ, Hajage D, et al. ECMO for severe ARDS: systematic review and individual patient data meta-analysis. Intensive Care Med 2020;46(11):2048–57.
70. Duan EH, Adhikari NKJ, D'Aragon F, et al. Management of acute respiratory distress syndrome and refractory hypoxemia. a multicenter observational study. Ann Am Thorac Soc 2017;14(12):1818–26.

Basic Modes of Mechanical Ventilation

Jared Ward, DO, MPH[a],*, Christopher Noel, MD[b]

KEYWORDS

- Mechanical ventilation • Ventilator modes • Ventilator management

KEY POINTS

- Respiratory failure requiring mechanical ventilation is common; emergency medicine providers must have expertise in ventilator management.
- Ventilators overcome resistance and compliance of the respiratory system to deliver gas flow. The relative contribution of each is easily measured and can help guide management.
- There is no perfect mode of mechanical ventilation. Each has its strengths and weaknesses and can be adapted to most clinical scenarios. The best mode is often the one that providers and staff are most familiar with.

INTRODUCTION

Emergency medicine (EM) providers are responsible for caring for a broad range of critically ill patients in acute, uncertain states of disease. Many of these patients require invasive mechanical ventilation for respiratory support and can spend prolonged periods of time under the care of EM providers.

With this responsibility, EM providers must have expertise in ventilator management. Yet, surveys indicate limited education and comfort with ventilator management.[1,2] Certainly, there is an opportunity for improvement.

This article aims to bridge the gap by providing an overview of ventilator management with an emphasis on modes, patient–ventilator interactions, and troubleshooting.

GOALS AND GENERAL PRINCIPLES OF MECHANICAL VENTILATION
Goals

The primary goals of mechanical ventilation are to provide physiologic support while minimizing harm. To this end, mechanical ventilation is used to maintain adequate

a Critical Care, Inspira Health Network, Inspira Medical Center Vineland, 1505 West Sherman Avenue, Vineland, NJ 08360, USA; b Division of Critical Care, Cooper University Health Care, Cooper Medical School of Rowan University, Cooper University Hospital, One Cooper Plaza, D429, Camden, NJ 08103, USA
* Corresponding author.
E-mail address: WardJ@ihn.org

Emerg Med Clin N Am 40 (2022) 473–488
https://doi.org/10.1016/j.emc.2022.05.003
0733-8627/22/© 2022 Elsevier Inc. All rights reserved.

emed.theclinics.com

gas exchange while minimizing harm due to excessive pressure, volume, and cyclic deformation of the lung. Like many critical interventions, it is supportive; it does not fix the underlying process that warrants its use.

Respiratory Mechanics

Mechanical ventilation provides respiratory support by generating positive pressure gas flow into a patient's lungs during inspiration and allowing for passive expiration. In passive or paralyzed patients, inspiration will be entirely controlled by the ventilator. In patients with respiratory drive, the inspiratory gas flow will occur as the result of patient effort and ventilator work.[3]

To deliver breaths, ventilators pressurize gas to overcome resistance to gas flow (from the ventilator tubing, endotracheal tube, and airways) and the elastic recoil of the lungs and surrounding structures. More simply, the pressure needed to inflate the lung is determined by the *resistance* and *compliance* of the respiratory system. Higher pressures are required when resistance increases, compliance worsens (the respiratory system becomes stiffer as indicated by a smaller change in volume per unit change in pressure), or both occur.

Understanding where the problem lies—high resistance or poor compliance—can help identify the initial cause of respiratory failure or sudden decompensation on the ventilator and guide management accordingly. Common causes for high resistance and poor compliance are shown in **Fig. 1**.

Expiration is a passive process that results from the pressure gradient between higher pressure in the alveoli and lower pressure at the ventilator. Importantly, ventilators can apply a positive end-expiratory pressure (PEEP) to lessen this pressure gradient and prevent excessive lung collapse.

Defining a Breath

The amount and timing of gas flow are determined by the inputs to the ventilator. Providers specify when a ventilator breath will occur, how it will be delivered (eg, an

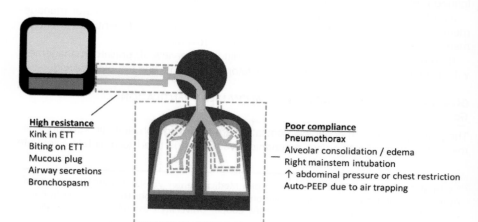

High resistance
Kink in ETT
Biting on ETT
Mucous plug
Airway secretions
Bronchospasm

Poor compliance
Pneumothorax
Alveolar consolidation / edema
Right mainstem intubation
↑ abdominal pressure or chest restriction
Auto-PEEP due to air trapping

Fig. 1. Common causes for high airway resistance and poor compliance. Areas of the respiratory circuit affecting resistance include the ventilator tubing, endotracheal tube, and airways to the level of the bronchioles. Areas of the respiratory circuit affecting compliance include the lung parenchyma (alveoli), pleural space, chest wall, abdomen, and anything external to the chest wall that exerts collapsing force on the alveoli.

applied pressure or flow rate), and when it will end via the trigger, control, and cycling variables.[3,4]

- *Trigger*: The trigger variable determines when inspiration occurs. This is specified as time (since the last breath) or either pressure or flow to detect when a patient makes an inspiratory effort. Whether pressure or flow serves as the trigger for patient-initiated breaths is rarely of clinical importance.
- *Control (or limit)*: The control variable determines how a ventilator delivers a breath. It is either flow or pressure. With flow, a breath is delivered at a specific flow rate (eg, 60 L per min). With pressure, the ventilator maintains a specific pressure during inspiration, and flow occurs as a result of the pressure differential between the ventilator and the patient's lungs.

The control variable must be either flow *or* pressure. It is impossible to specify both at the same time.

- *Cycling*: The cycling variable determines when inspiration ends and expiration begins. It is either time, volume, or flow—with flow specifying a percentage of peak inspiratory flow when inspiration ends.

The combination of trigger, control, and cycling variables, among others,[5] helps define specific ventilator modes.

COMMON MODES OF MECHANICAL VENTILATION

A ventilator mode is the set of rules, or algorithms, used to deliver breaths throughout the respiratory cycle and is the first selection made when initiating mechanical ventilation.

The names for ventilator modes and the specific algorithms used to define them can vary across different ventilator manufacturers but generally work in the same way. The most common ventilator modes are forms of volume control (VC)—also known as volume assist control, pressure control (PC)—also known as pressure assist control, and pressure support (PS). These are sufficient for most, if not all, clinical scenarios. Other modes rely on more complex algorithms and include pressure-regulated VC (PRVC), synchronized intermittent mandatory ventilation (SIMV), and airway pressure release ventilation (APRV).

The trigger, control, and cycling variables used for each mode are shown in **Table 1**.

Volume Control

In VC ventilation, the same prespecified tidal volume is delivered with each inspiratory cycle, regardless of whether the breath is time or patient triggered (**Fig. 2**).

The key provider settings include:

- Flow rate*
- Tidal volume
- Respiratory rate
- PEEP
- Fraction of inspired oxygen (FiO_2)

* Depending on the ventilator, the user will input either the flow rate and tidal volume or the inspiratory time and tidal volume.

In VC ventilation, pressure is not controlled. It is a dependent variable determined by airway resistance and lung compliance. As resistance increases or compliance worsens, the flow will remain constant, and pressures will rise.

Table 1 Variables defining common ventilator modes			
Mode	**Trigger**	**Control**	**Cycling**
Volume control	Time or patient initiated (pressure or flow)	Flow	Volume
Pressure control	Time or patient initiated	Pressure	Time
Pressure support	Patient initiated	Pressure	Flow
Pressure regulated volume control	Time or patient initiated	Pressure	Time

SIMV and APRV are not included as they are beyond the scope of this article.

Advantages of VC ventilation include guaranteed tidal volumes, stable minute ventilation, and the ability to specify a flow rate, which could be advantageous in a setting of high airway resistance.

Disadvantages are that injurious pressures may be generated in the setting of worsening lung compliance or high resistance.

Pressure Control

In PC ventilation, a constant inspiratory pressure is applied throughout inspiration, regardless of whether the ventilator or the patient initiates the breath (**Fig. 3**).

The key provider settings include:

- Inspiratory pressure*
- Inspiratory time
- Respiratory rate
- PEEP
- FiO_2

* Depending on the ventilator, the user will input either the total inspiratory pressure desired or the inspiratory pressure to be applied above PEEP.

In this mode, flow and resulting tidal volume are dependent variables and vary with changes in airway resistance and lung compliance.

One advantage of PC is that airway and pulmonary pressures never exceed the selected inspiratory pressure. Thus, the risk for barotrauma can be minimized. Another advantage is that patients control their inspiratory flow rate—air flow will increase in proportion to their inspiratory effort, improving patient comfort and minimizing patient–ventilator dyssynchrony.

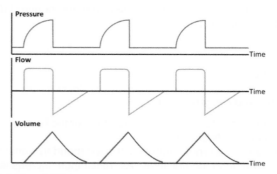

Fig. 2. Volume control waveforms.

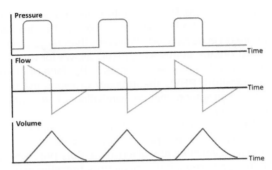

Fig. 3. Pressure control waveforms.

A disadvantage is that the delivered tidal volume can vary. As resistance decreases or compliance improves, the same pressure may lead to excessive tidal volumes. Alternatively, if resistance increases or compliance worsens, the same pressure will generate much smaller volumes and result in poor ventilation, carbon dioxide retention, and ventilatory failure.

Pressure-Regulated Volume Control

PRVC is a mode of mechanical ventilation that uses an adaptive targeting scheme to automatically adjust the inspiratory pressure to achieve a specified tidal volume[5] (**Fig. 4**).

The key provider settings include:

- Target tidal volume
- Inspiratory time
- Respiratory rate
- PEEP
- FiO_2

The commonly used name for this mode, PRVC, is misleading. Flow and volume are not controlled. Pressure is the control variable, and flow varies with changes in airway resistance, lung compliance, and patient effort.

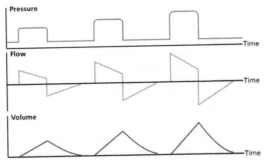

Fig. 4. Pressure-regulated volume control waveforms. In this example, the ventilator automatically increases the inspiratory pressure to achieve the desired tidal volume.

To achieve a target tidal volume, PRVC monitors the tidal volume resulting from the applied inspiratory pressure. If the tidal volume is higher than the target, the applied pressure for the next breath is decreased. If it is less than target, the applied pressure is increased for the next breath. In this way, PRVC allows for breath-by-breath pressure adjustments to achieve the desired volumes in the face of changing resistance, compliance, and patient effort. PRVC theoretically provides the benefits of variable flow from PC with the guaranteed minute ventilation of VC without requiring the user to adjust the inspiratory pressure.

A disadvantage of PRVC is the potential for patient–ventilator dyssynchrony in patients with high respiratory drives. If a patient develops increased work of breathing and is generating large tidal volumes at a given inspiratory pressure, the adaptive targeting scheme will continue to reduce the inspiratory pressure with each subsequent breath. This results in less support from the ventilator and an increase in patient work of breathing.[6] PRVC should, therefore, be used in patients who have stable respiratory drives.

Pressure Support

PS ventilation is a mode of mechanical ventilation whereby the inspiratory pressure is controlled, but all breaths, flow, and inspiratory time are determined by the patient (**Fig. 5**).

The provider settings include:

- Inspiratory pressure
- Percentage of peak inspiratory flow rate to terminate inspiration
- PEEP
- FiO_2

In PS, there is no set respiratory rate or inspiratory time. All breaths are triggered by the patient, and inspiration continues until the inspiratory flow decays below a selected value (eg, 30% of peak flow).

PS is often used in weaning patients off mechanical ventilation as patients control the inspiratory flow rate, duration of inspiration, and respiratory rate. Patients with a depressed respiratory drive, high oxygen consumption, or elevated airway resistance are not appropriate candidates for PS that generally excludes its use in the emergency department.

EVALUATING RESPIRATORY MECHANICS
Evaluating Respiratory Mechanics in Different Modes

Changes in resistance and compliance manifest differently with different modes of mechanical ventilation.

Volume control

In VC ventilation, increased resistance or worsening compliance or both result in increases in pressure. The two scenarios can be differentiated by comparing the maximum pressure during inspiration or peak pressure, and the pressure required to keep the lung inflated once the inspiratory flow has stopped or plateau pressure.

The peak pressure is simply the highest pressure observed on the pressure versus time displayed on the ventilator. The plateau pressure is measured by performing an inspiratory hold maneuver, where the ventilator ceases airflow at the end of inspiration and measures the pressure in the respiratory circuit. Because the lungs are fully inflated and exhalation has not yet occurred, this represents the total pressure in the lungs, inclusive of PEEP, at a specified volume.

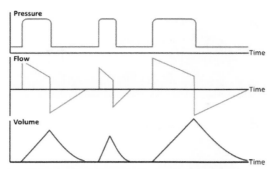

Fig. 5. Pressure support waveforms, showing fixed inspiratory pressure but varying inspiratory time, respiratory rate, and tidal volume based on patient effort.

A large differential between the peak and plateau pressure will be observed when the limiting factor to gas delivery is resistance to airflow (eg, obstructed airway and normal lungs). A small differential will occur when the limiting factor is the compliance of the respiratory systems (eg, widely patent airways, diffuse alveolar disease). This is shown in the pressure versus time curve in **Fig. 6**.

Pressure control or pressure support

In PC and PS ventilation, the inspiratory pressure is fixed at the value set by the operator. Therefore, higher resistance or worsening compliance will both cause a decrease in observed tidal volumes without a way to reliably differentiate between these two scenarios.

Pressure-regulated volume control

As an adaptive mode, PRVC varies the inspiratory pressure based on the mechanics of the respiratory system. Higher resistance or worsening compliance causes the ventilator to increase the inspiratory pressure to achieve the target tidal volume. The difference between the peak and plateau pressures can be measured with an inspiratory hold, just as in VC.

Auto-Positive End-Expiratory Pressure

A special cause of worsening respiratory compliance occurs when patients do not fully exhale before the initiation of the next breath. Air becomes trapped in the lungs such that there is retained pressure in excess of the applied-PEEP or auto-PEEP.

As auto-PEEP builds, higher and higher inspiratory pressures are required to deliver a desired tidal volume. Left unchecked, this can lead to pneumothorax or compromised venous return and cardiovascular collapse.

Auto-PEEP is measured using an end-expiratory hold maneuver. An end-expiratory hold maneuver stops airflow at the end of expiration and evaluates the pressure at this time. This pressure represents the sum of the retained pressure (auto-PEEP) and applied pressure (PEEP) and is referred to as the total-PEEP. Normally, the total-PEEP will equal the applied-PEEP. When air trapping occurs, the total-PEEP measurement will be higher than the applied-PEEP due to auto-PEEP.

The flow versus time display can often give a clue to air trapping and the presence of auto-PEEP when it does not return to the zero baselines by the end of expiration (representing incomplete exhalation). However, relying on this can miss significant auto-PEEP, so an end-expiratory hold maneuver should be performed.

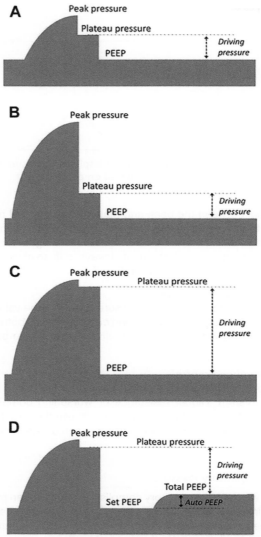

Fig. 6. (*A*) Normal pressure versus time curve in volume control ventilation. (*B*) Elevated peak airway pressures without elevation of plateau pressure secondary to increased resistance. (*C*) Elevated peak and plateau pressures due to poor compliance. (*D*) Elevated peak and plateau pressures due to auto-PEEP from air trapping.

Auto-PEEP can occur because of severe bronchospasm or inappropriate ventilator settings or both. Strategies to reduce auto-PEEP include decreasing respiratory rate and shortening the inspiratory time to lengthen expiration (**Fig. 7**).

Driving Pressure

Driving pressure is defined as the difference between the plateau pressure and the total-PEEP. Conceptually, it represents the pressure above the PEEP required to

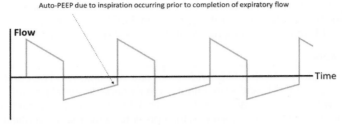

Auto-PEEP due to inspiration occurring prior to completion of expiratory flow

Fig. 7. Flow-time graph indicating auto-PEEP.

keep the lung inflated to a chosen tidal volume. The static compliance of the lung is equal to the tidal volume divided by the driving pressure.

$$static\ compliance = \frac{tidal\ volume}{plateau\ pressure - total\ PEEP} = \frac{tidal\ volume}{driving\ pressure}$$

Therefore, driving pressure is inversely proportional with pulmonary compliance. Less compliant, or "stiffer," lungs will require higher driving pressures to achieve the same tidal volume.

Driving pressures strongly correlates with mortality in patients with ARDS, with values < 15 cm H_2O thought to be protective.[7]

When to Measure Respiratory Mechanics

The inspiratory and expiratory hold maneuvers are key to understanding a patient's respiratory mechanics. However, they should only be measured when a patient is passive and compliant with the ventilator. Otherwise, a patient's negative inspiratory efforts can lead to an underestimate of the plateau pressure and an overestimation of lung compliance. Importantly, paralytics should not be given for the sole purpose of getting accurate measurements.

INITIAL SETTINGS
Tidal Volume

The initial tidal volume should be 6 to 8 cc/kg predicted body weight for most patients and adjusted as needed to ensure that the plateau pressure is ≤ 30 cm H_2O.[8,9]

Patients without ARDS may tolerate higher tidal volumes of 10 mL/kg predicted body weight without ill effect.[10] However, ARDS is often underrecognized, so targeting 6 to 8 cc/kg predicted body weight for most patients, and certainly less than 6 cc/kg predicted body weight in patients with ARDS is advised.[11–13]

If using PC, the inspiratory pressure should be set to achieve these targets with an ongoing patient reassessment to avoid excessive tidal volumes.

Positive End-Expiratory Pressure

A PEEP should be set for all patients to minimize traumatic opening and closing of alveoli, known as atelectotrauma.[13]

Higher PEEP values (≥5 mmHg) should be selected in the setting of ARDS to minimize atelectotrauma and intrapulmonary shunt and pulmonary edema to decrease venous return and reduce afterload.[14]

PEEP optimization is a complex topic without a consensus approach. A straightforward approach is to set PEEP according to the PEEP/FiO$_2$ tables used by ARDS

Network investigators, which showed a decreased mortality with low tidal volume ventilation in ARDS.[9] Another strategy is to set PEEP to maximize compliance by setting the PEEP at the level that results in the lowest driving pressure.

Respiratory Rate

The initial respiratory rate should provide adequate ventilation and be comfortable for the patient. The 14 to 18 breaths per minute is reasonable for most patients. However, for patients with metabolic acidosis (eg, salicylate overdose), the respiratory rate should be increased to match or exceed their pre-intubation minute ventilation. Failing to do so may worsen acidosis and can precipitate complications, such as cardiac arrest.[14]

Fraction of Inspired Oxygen

FiO_2 should be initially set at 100% in the setting of hypoxia and rapidly weaned to target a PaO_2 of 60 to 100 mmHg or SpO_2 92% to 96%[15,16] (**Fig. 8**).

COMMON TROUBLESHOOTING SCENARIOS
Elevated Peak Airway Pressures

The plateau pressure should be measured with an inspiratory hold maneuver to differentiate between high resistance (large peak-plateau pressure differential) and poor compliance (small differential) scenarios, as previously discussed (**Fig. 9**).

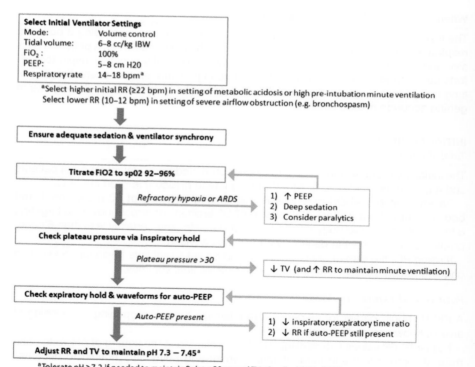

Fig. 8. Algorithm for initiating mechanical ventilation. BPM, breaths per minute; H_2O, water; IBW, ideal body weight; RR, respiratory rate.

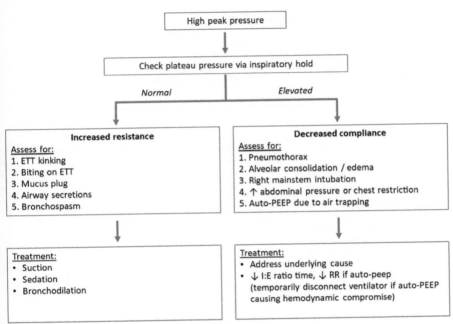

Fig. 9. Management algorithm for addressing elevated peak airway pressure.

Dyssynchrony

Patient–ventilator dyssynchrony arises from mechanical ventilation mimicking, but not matching, a patient's spontaneous respiratory mechanics. It is common and increases work of breathing, patient discomfort and reduces the effectiveness of ventilatory support[17] (**Fig. 10**).

Dyssynchrony is important to recognize and can easily be identified on ventilator waveforms. There are three major types of patient–ventilator dyssynchrony: flow, trigger, and cycle.

Flow dyssynchrony, or flow starvation, occurs in VC ventilation when flow does not meet patient demands. On a pressure versus time curve, the normal convex shape becomes concave, and the observed airway pressure decreases. Flow starvation can be fixed by increasing the flow rate or changing to PC ventilation (**Fig.11**).

Trigger dyssynchrony refers to when too many or too few patient-triggered breaths are delivered. The most common types of trigger dyssynchrony are ineffective triggering, auto-triggering, or double triggering and can occur in any of the modes previously discussed.

Ineffective triggering occurs when the ventilator does not deliver a breath after a patient inspiratory effort. It is most commonly because of inappropriate flow or pressure trigger settings. The clinician observes a negative deflection in the flow or pressure versus time curve (indicating a patient inspiratory effort) not immediately followed by a ventilator breath. Conversely, auto-triggering occurs when ventilator breaths are delivered without patient inspiratory effort. This is commonly caused by condensation in the ventilator tubing, vigorous cardiac activity, or circuit leaks when the flow or pressure trigger sensitivity is too sensitive. Adjusting the trigger sensitivity usually resolves ineffective and auto-triggering. Both scenarios are depicted in **Fig. 12**.

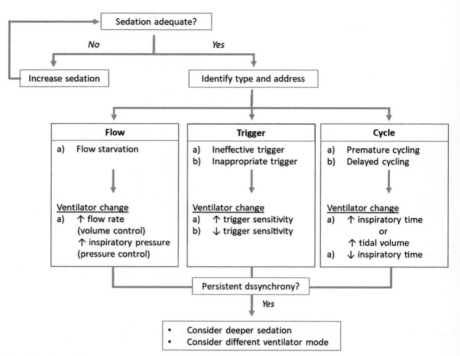

Fig. 10. Algorithm to manage common forms of ventilator dyssynchrony.

Cycle dyssynchrony occurs when inspiratory gas flow stops prematurely or continues into a patient's natural expiratory phase. An example of a patient's expiratory phase beginning before the end of the ventilator delivered breath is shown in **Fig. 13**. In PC, VC, and PRVC, this can be fixed by shortening or lengthening the inspiratory time, respectively. In PS, this is addressed by reducing or increasing the percentage of peak flow when cycling from inspiration to expiration occurs (**Fig. 14**).

Double triggering occurs when a second breath is triggered immediately after the first and is commonly referred to as "stacked breaths." This most often occurs in VC, PC, or PRVC due to a form of cycle dyssynchrony known as premature cycling, where the patient's respiratory drive exceeds the ventilator-delivered volume or inspiratory time. Increasing sedation, tidal volumes or flow, inspiratory pressure, or inspiratory time can fix this form of double triggering.

Leak

A leak should be suspected if the measured exhaled volume does not equal the inspiratory volume, or the volume versus time curve does not return to baseline before the next breath.

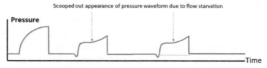

Fig. 11. Pressure–time graph showing flow starvation.

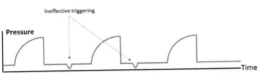

Fig. 12. Pressure–time graph showing ineffective triggering whereby the ventilator does not deliver a breath despite a negative pressure inspiratory effort by the patient due to inappropriate trigger sensitivity settings.

PITFALLS
Inadequate Analgosedation

Attempting to troubleshoot respiratory mechanics or dyssynchrony without adequate analgosedation will result in inaccurate measurements and misleading waveforms. Therefore, ensure adequate analgosedation before measuring the plateau pressure, checking for auto-PEEP, dramatically changing settings, or switching modes.

Assuming a Ventilator Mode Will Fix Poor Respiratory Mechanics

As discussed, ventilator settings should be chosen to target a plateau pressure less than 30 cm H_2O and driving pressure less than 15 cm H_2O. When pulmonary compliance is extremely poor, however, these goals may not be possible. Switching modes will not change the situation and may be harmful. For example, switching from VC to PC to achieve a lower inspiratory pressure will result in smaller and possibly inadequate volumes and hypoventilation.

Failing to Reassess

As with any intervention, reassessment is the key. Airway pressures, tidal volumes, oxygenation, and synchrony should be frequently monitored, particularly if the patient's conditions change.

DISCUSSION

Mechanically ventilated patients are common in the ED. Unfortunately, these patients sometimes remain in the ED for prolonged periods of time, with resulting in increased duration of mechanical ventilation, longer ICU length of stay, and higher mortality.[18–20]

Early ventilator management represents an opportunity for improvement. Indeed, less than half of ED patients with identified ARDS received low tidal volume ventilation in one observational study.[21] This is particularly concerning as ventilator-induced lung injury can occur in as little as 20 minutes.[22] Patients without ARDS may also be at risk as large tidal volumes within the first 48 hours of care have been associated with subsequent development of ARDS.[23] Fortunately, best practice strategies can be successfully implemented in the ED to decrease mortality, duration of ventilation, and hospital length of stay.[24]

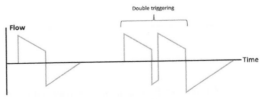

Fig. 13. Flow-time graph showing double-triggering.

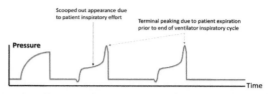

Fig. 14. Pressure versus time curve in volume control showing early scooping and a late spike in pressure as a patient makes a vigorous inspiratory effort and then attempts to exhale when the ventilator breath is still being delivered.

Education is another opportunity for improvement. Commonly, ventilated patients are managed by physicians without subspecialty training, and there is evidence of insufficient mechanical ventilation education and management for this group.[25] Furthermore, a survey of EM attending physicians showed many received 3 hours or less ventilator training over the last year and many identified a respiratory therapist as being primarily responsible for ventilator management. Higher ventilator management scores correlated with prior emphasis on mechanical ventilation in the physician's residency training; however, a previous study of EM residents reported an infrequent exposure to and a little education on mechanical ventilation.[1,2]

All of these data highlight several important findings. There is increasing importance for EM providers to understand various modes of mechanical ventilation, initiate best practice ventilator settings early, and identify and treat complications of the ventilator when they arise. Understanding why changes in resistance and compliance occur, how they are represented graphically, and where they correlate anatomically is paramount to troubleshooting.

SUMMARY

Acute respiratory failure requiring invasive mechanical ventilation is a common presentation in the emergency department. EM providers can further improve care for these patients by understanding common modes of mechanical ventilation, recognizing changes in respiratory mechanics, and tailoring ventilator settings and therapies accordingly.

CLINICS CARE POINTS

- Respiratory failure requiring mechanical ventilation is common; emergency medicine providers must have expertise in ventilator management.
- Ventilators overcome resistance and compliance of the respiratory system to deliver gas flow. The relative contribution of each is easily measured and can help guide management.
- There is no perfect mode of mechanical ventilation. Each has its strengths and weaknesses and can be adapted to most clinical scenarios. The best mode is often the one that providers and staff are most familiar with.

DISCLOSURE

Dr J. Ward and Dr C. Noel have no financial or commercial conflicts of interest to report. No funding was provided for this project.

REFERENCES

1. Wilcox SR, Todd TA, Trout TD, et al. Emergency medicine residents' knowledge of mechanical ventilation. J Emerg Med 2015;48(4):481–91.
2. Wilcox SR, Trout TD, Schneider JI, et al. Academic emergency medicine physicians' knowledge of mechanical ventilation. West J Emerg Med 2016;17(3):271.
3. Chatburn, R.L. Engineering principles applied to mechanical ventilation. in Proceedings of the 25th Annual International Conference of the IEEE Engineering in Medicine and Biology Society (IEEE Cat. No. 03CH37439). 17-21 September 2003:Cancun, Mexico. IEEE.
4. Kapadia F. Mechanical ventilation: simplifying the terminology. Postgrad Med J 1998;74(872):330–5.
5. Chatburn RL, El-Khatib M, Mireles-Cabodevila E. A taxonomy for mechanical ventilation: 10 fundamental maxims. Respir Care 2014;59(11):1747–63.
6. Singh G, Chien C, Patel S. Pressure regulated volume control (PRVC): set it and forget it? Respir Med case Rep 2020;29:100822.
7. Amato MB, Meade MO, Slutsky AS, et al. Driving pressure and survival in the acute respiratory distress syndrome. N Engl J Med 2015;372(8):747–55.
8. Lellouche F, Lipes J. Prophylactic protective ventilation: lower tidal volumes for all critically ill patients? Intensive Care Med 2013;39(1):6–15.
9. Network ARDS. Ventilation with lower tidal volumes as compared with traditional tidal volumes for acute lung injury and the acute respiratory distress syndrome. N Engl J Med 2000;342(18):1301–8.
10. Simonis FD, Neto AS, Binnekade JM, et al. Effect of a low vs intermediate tidal volume strategy on ventilator-free days in intensive care unit patients without ARDS: a randomized clinical trial. JAMA 2018;320(18):1872–80.
11. Fröhlich S, Murphy N, Doolan A, et al. Acute respiratory distress syndrome: underrecognition by clinicians. J Crit Care 2013;28(5):663–8.
12. Bellani G, Laffey JG, Pham T, et al. Epidemiology, patterns of care, and mortality for patients with acute respiratory distress syndrome in intensive care units in 50 countries. JAMA 2016;315(8):788–800.
13. Chen J-T, Gong M. Universal low tidal volume: early initiation of low tidal volume ventilation in patients with and without ARDS. In: Jean-Louis Vincent eds. Annual update in intensive care and emergency medicine 2019 Switzerland AG: Springer; 2019. p. 47–58.
14. Carpio ALM, Mora JI. Ventilator management Treasure Island: StatPearls; 2021.
15. Angus DC. Oxygen Therapy for the Critically Ill. N Engl J Med. 2020;382(11):1054-1056.
16.. Siemieniuk RA, Chu DK, Kim LH, et al. Oxygen therapy for acutely ill medical patients: a clinical practice guideline. Bmj 2018;363.
17. Nilsestuen JO, Hargett KD. Using ventilator graphics to identify patient-ventilator asynchrony. Respir Care 2005;50(2):202–34.
18. Easter BD, Fischer C, Fisher J. The use of mechanical ventilation in the ED. Am J Emerg Med 2012;30(7):1183–8.
19. Mohr NM, et al. Boarding of critically ill patients in the emergency department. J Am CollEmerg Physicians Open 2020;1(4):423–31.
20. Singer AJ, Thode HC, Viccelio P, et al. The association between length of emergency department boarding and mortality. AcadEmerg Med 2011;18(12):1324–9.
21. Fuller BM, Mohr NM, Miller CN, et al. Mechanical ventilation and ARDS in the ED: a multicenter, observational, prospective, cross-sectional study. Chest 2015; 148(2):365–74.

22. Hoegl S, Boost KA, Flondor M, et al. Short-term exposure to high-pressure venti-lation leads to pulmonary biotrauma and systemic inflammation in the rat. Int J Mol Med 2008;21(4):513–9.
23. Gajic O, Frutos-Vivar F, Esteban A, et al. Ventilator settings as a risk factor for acute respiratory distress syndrome in mechanically ventilated patients. Intensive Care Med 2005;31(7):922–6.
24. Fuller BM, Ferguson IT, Mohr NM, et al. Lung-protective ventilation initiated in the emergency department (LOV-ED): a quasi-experimental, before-after trial. Ann Emerg Med 2017;70(3):406–18.e4.
25. Sweigart JR, Aymond D, Burger A, et al. Characterizing hospitalist practice and perceptions of critical care delivery. J Hosp Med 2018;13(1):6. Available at: www.journalofhospitalmedicine.com.

Airway Pressure Release Ventilation

A Field Guide for the Emergency Physician

Rory Spiegel, MD[a,b,*], Max Hockstein, MD[a,b,1]

KEYWORDS

• APRV • ARDS • Hypoxemia

KEY POINTS

- Airway pressure release ventilation (APRV) uses high airway pressures to recruit and maintain lung volumes.
- The goals of APRV are to return patients lung volumes to functional residual capacity and to promote safe spontaneous breathing.
- APRV should be viewed as continuous positive airway pressure with release volumes intended to augment ventilation.

INTRODUCTION

The goal of mechanical ventilation (MV) is to provide a critically ill patient with physiologic gas exchange, whereas minimizing iatrogenesis and facilitating ventilator liberation.[1] Substantial effort has been placed into defining safe MV parameters for patients with and without acute respiratory distress syndrome (ARDS).[2,3] Owing, in part, to dedicated study, the mortality of ARDS has improved during the past several decades.[4] Salient discoveries in the management of ARDS include the institution of lung protective ventilation and prone positioning.[2,5] Benefits common to both of these interventions include the avoidance of overdistension of healthy alveoli and the maintenance of lung volumes.

CASE PRESENTATION

A 49 year-old woman is admitted to the ED for pneumonia. During her ED course, she becomes more hypoxic requiring endotracheal intubation. Unfortunately, there are no ICU beds available. A chest X-ray demonstrates bilateral, patchy infiltrates with

---

[a] Department of Emergency Medicine, MedStar Washington Hospital Center; [b] Department of Critical Care, MedStar Washington Hospital Center
[1] Present address: 524 8th Street Northwest, Washington, DC 20002.
* Corresponding author. 1423 33rd Street Northwest, Washington, DC 20007.
E-mail address: rspiegs@gmail.com

Emerg Med Clin N Am 40 (2022) 489–501
https://doi.org/10.1016/j.emc.2022.05.004
0733-8627/22/© 2022 Elsevier Inc. All rights reserved.

emed.theclinics.com

adequate positioning of the endotracheal tube. The patient was placed on volume control ventilation with a rate of 24, a tidal volume of 500 mL, an Fio_2 of 0.8, and a PEEP of +10 cm H_2O. A plateau pressure was measured at 28 cm H_2O. An ABG reveals a pH of 7.34, a Pco_2 of 57 mm Hg, and a Po_2 of 50 mm Hg.

ACUTE RESPIRATORY DISTRESS SYNDROME PHYSIOLOGY

ARDS is a process, which reduces the size of the functional lung resulting in a "baby lung."[6] The "baby lung" is the island(s) of healthy lung parenchyma adjacent to the parenchyma affected by ARDS. MV exposes both the affected and unaffected lung to the set ventilation parameters; however, the 2 parenchymal areas accommodate gas flow differently. Delivered gas is directed preferentially to the alveoli with the lowest alveolar pressures, the unaffected regions of the lung are subjected to higher delivered volumes leading to overdistension and potential worsening of lung injury.[7–9]

Although ARDS has expansive causes and complex physiologic implications, in the ED, it is easiest to think of it as a portion of the lung as derecruited and, therefore, not participating in ventilation. Although ventilation is preferentially distributed to the nonaffected areas of the lung, perfusion is more homogenously distributed throughout the lung. Perfusion of nonaerated lung leads to blood passing through the lung without the opportunity to participate in gas exchange, a phenomenon known as shunt. Shunt is reflected by hypoexmia that seems to be refractory to the application of supplemental oxygen.

The more severe the ARDS, the larger the portion of affected lung. Consequently, the larger the portion of lung affected, the worse the hypoxemia. As the definition of functional residual capacity (FRC) is defined as "the volume of gas in the lung after a normal expiration," in patients with ARDS, the patient's FRC is significantly reduced.[10]

Alveolar recruitment does not follow a commonly conceived "inflated or deflated" paradigm. Instead, the lung exhibits viscoelastic behavior. Alveoli both dynamically resist volume changes over time (a property of viscosity) and quickly assume their derecruited form when the stressor is removed (a property of elasticity). Therefore, the lung does not instantaneously change its volume in response to the application of pressure; rather, it will do so over time. Given these physiologic properties, it stands that one must apply pressure-over-time in order to rerecruit lung and restore FRC. This is why tidal pressures do nothing to recruit lung and the application of PEEP is necessary to optimize alveolar recruitment and prevent derecruitment by raising mean airway pressures.

The goals of MV in patients with ARDS are 2-fold. First, to ensure the volumes of gas delivered is appropriate for the size of the lung participating in ventilation. Second, to restore patients' FRC, whereby increasing the portion of the lung, which is participating in ventilation.

AIRWAY PRESSURE RELEASE VENTILATION

Airway pressure release ventilation (APRV) is a mode of ventilation that uses high airway pressures to recruit alveoli and maintain patients' physiologic lung volumes. The goal of this mode of ventilation is 2-fold: first, to maintain patients as close to their FRC as possible and second, to promote safe spontaneous breathing. Although there are several unique names for the mode by different manufacturers (**Table 1**), all function similarly.

APRV should essentially be viewed as continuous positive airway pressure (CPAP), with intermittent releases of that pressure to metabolically support patients who are

Table 1
Airway pressure release ventilation mode names by different manufacturers

Manufacturer	Mode Name
Drager	PC-APRV
CareScape	APRV
Hamilton Galileo	APRV
Puritan Benett	840: BILEVEL 980: APRV
Servo	Bi-Vent
Vela	APRV/BiPhasic

Abbreviations: APRV, airway pressure release ventilation.

incapable of managing their ventilatory load. Imagine for a moment, a patient presents to you in the emergency department in respiratory distress. This patient was breathing comfortably with normal respiratory mechanics just a few days prior. Whatever respiratory insult that caused this presentation is simply due to worsening compliance of the lung parenchyma resulting in reduced resting lung volumes less than FRC. The patient's respiratory muscles are working just as well as they did previously, only now they have to work harder to manage the same volume of CO_2 production.

If one could restore the patient back to their previous lung volumes with the use of PEEP, then potentially the patient could more comfortably breathe on their own. The classic example of this is a patient presenting to the ED with pulmonary edema due to congestive heart failure. These patients typically have relatively normal respiratory muscles and have respiratory distress due to the increased extravascular lung water leading to a heavy lung resulting in reduced lung volumes. The use of noninvasive positive pressure ventilation is so effective in this patient population because it allows for the clinician to reestablish normal lung volumes using a noninvasive form of PEEP (expiratory positive airway pressure). Rapid restoration of normal lung volumes is readily obtainable due to the relative swift recruitability of patients with cardiogenic pulmonary edema. This is why most of these patients are managed noninvasively, not requiring invasive MV.

Unfortunately, most forms of respiratory distress are due to underlying disease processes that are not as easily recruitable as cardiogenic pulmonary edema. Moreover, although the application of PEEP will often restore normal lung volumes, it does so in a slow fashion. Given the reluctant nature of lung recruitment of an injured lung, it is not feasible or safe to expect patients to manage their own ventilation. During this period of recruitment, until the patient can safely manage their own ventilatory needs with spontaneous breathing, APRV uses what is known as a release volume to achieve its ventilatory ends.

A release volume consists of a momentary release of CPAP causing a rapid decrease in airway pressure and the subsequent exhalation of CO_2 (**Fig. 1**). What makes APRV different from other forms of inverse ratio ventilation (IRV) (where inspiratory-to-expiratory ratio exceeds conventional targets) is that this release volume is precisely controlled to encourage offloading of CO_2 while limiting the actual change in lung volumes. In fact, we would argue that it is the control of the release volumes, which endow APRV with its unique properties. Although there are many other aspects of APRV that will be discussed in this review, unless clinicians are mindful of preventing derecruitment during the release phases, then the benefits associated with this mode of ventilation are likely to be lost and additional injury may occur.

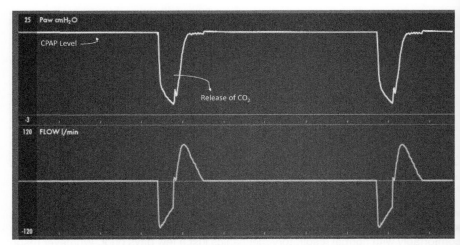

Fig. 1. APRV pressure and flow scalars demonstrating 2 phases: CPAP phase and release phase. During CPAP level, alveolar recruitment is accomplished and during the release phase, CO_2 is released.

    As patients recruit and lungs approach the patient's natural lung volumes, their ability to breathe spontaneously and manage their own ventilatory needs improves. As such, the need to augment their ventilatory efforts decreases, and release breaths are required less frequently. Eventually, patients are able to fully support their ventilatory needs and no longer require any release breaths to maintain normal CO_2 levels. Now, the patients can be "stretched" to CPAP (**Fig. 2**).

    When discussing the literature examining the efficacy of APRV, it is important to differentiate IRV from APRV. IRV is a pressure-controlled mode of ventilation that spends most of the respiratory cycle in the inspiratory phase and, as a consequence,

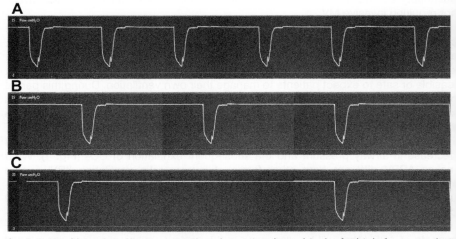

Fig. 2. APRV liberation. Note progressive elongation (stretching) of T-high from panels A through C. (A) initial APRV setup. (B) APRV maintenance. (C) Approaching evolution to CPAP.

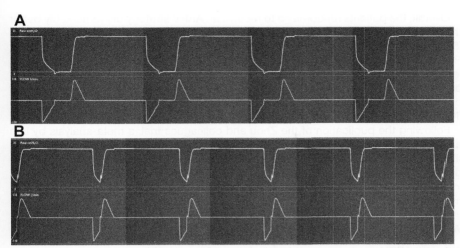

Fig. 3. (*A*) Note excessive timing of T-low resulting in full exhalation manifested by flow scalar returning to baseline between CPAP phases. (*B*) Appropriate timing of T-low resulting in trapping.

a far smaller portion in the expiratory phase. What differentiates APRV from the more general IRV, is the expiratory phase is titrated to the patient's individual lung compliance, ensuring that the expiratory time is limited to 75% of patient's peak expiratory flow rate (PEFR; **Fig. 3**). In other words, when compared with breaths delivered in traditional modes of MV, APRV does not allow for a "full" exhalation (ie, 100% of PEFR) during the timed release.

Jain and colleagues noted that there is an inconsistency among the studies claiming to study APRV because many of them use a fixed expiratory time (fixed APRV), not titrating based on the patient's individual lung mechanics (personalized APRV), thus allowing many of the patients to fully exhale.[11] When all studies claiming to examine APRV are examined in totality, there does not seem to be a benefit in its use but when the studies that do not mandate a titration of the time low (T-low) in concordance with the patient's lung mechanics are excluded, APRV was found to be superior to more traditional modes of ventilation, leading to a decrease in the time spent on MV as well as mortality.

Probably, the most well-done RCT comparing APRV to LTV strategies using more traditional modes of ventilation is a trial published by Zhou and colleagues.[12] Published in Intensive Care Medicine in November of 2017, the authors enrolled patients presenting to a single center with hypoxic respiratory failure, requiring mechanical ventilatory support, who fulfilled the diagnostic criteria of ARDS according to the Berlin definition, a Pao_2/Fio_2 of less than 250, and were mechanically ventilated for less than 48 hours. Patients were randomized to receive either a traditional ARDSNet lung protective strategy (targeted tidal volume of 6 mL/kg predicted body weight using a volume assist mode of MV, PEEP levels determined by a PEEP-FiO_2 table and respiratory rates [RRs] titrated to limit hypercapnia and respiratory acidosis), or to APRV. Patients randomized to the APRV arm were placed on a pressure high (P-high) according to the plateau pressure that was obtained on their previous traditional volume control setting, a pressure low (P-low) of 0 to 5 cm H_2O, and a T-low titrated to the patients' intrinsic compliance.

Overall, the patients randomized to receive an APRV strategy did remarkably better than their low-tidal volume counterparts, boasting significantly fewer ventilator days (8 [5–14] vs 15 [7–22] P = .001), higher rate of successful extubation (66.2% vs 38.8% P = .001), and fewer tracheostomies (12.7% vs 29.9% P = .013). They also required less additional supportive measures including paralysis, recruitment maneuvers, and prone positioning. Moreover, although not statistically significant, the point estimate of both ICU mortality and hospital mortality trended strongly in favor of the APRV group (ICU mortality 19.7% vs 34.3% P = .053, hospital mortality 23.9% vs 37.3% P = .088).

Following the publication of the Zhou and colleagues trial, a meta-analysis by Lim and colleagues was published in Critical Care Medicine in 2019.[13] The authors identified 7 RCTs with a total of 412 patients admitted to the ICU for ARDS on MV and randomized to either APRV or a traditional mode of ventilation. The authors found an improvement in mortality in patients who received APRV compared with traditional modes of ventilation.

WHEN TO CONSIDER AIRWAY PRESSURE RELEASE VENTILATION?

Although APRV was once considered a "rescue" mode of MV, its early application in a patient's course has tangible benefits regarding lung mechanics and mortality. APRV has been examined across several clinical domains including ARDS from pneumonia, pulmonary contusions in the setting of trauma, and postcardiac surgery.[12,14,15] In the emergency department, APRV's primary role should be in patients with hypoxemia refractory to traditional modes of ventilation. For the sake of this document, we will consider refractory hypoxemia as an oxygen saturation less than 92% despite an Fio_2 of 1. Typically, cases of refractory hypoxemia in the ED are due to intrapulmonary shunting.[16]

Before using APRV in a patient with refractory hypoxemia, the clinician should endeavor to identify the type of shunt causing the hypoxemia. Clinicians will encounter 2 distinct types of intrapulmonary shunt leading to refractory hypoxemia, single or double lung shunt physiology.

Single lung shunt physiology occurs when the pathologic process is occurring in only one of the patient's lungs and leaves the contralateral side untouched. This can often be caused by lobar pneumonia, mucous plugging, atelectasis, and right mainstem intubation (**Fig. 4**A). Double lung shunt physiology occurs when the cause of the hypoxemia is more diffuse and affects bilateral lungs (**Fig. 4**B). This is often seen in multifocal pneumonia, pulmonary edema, ARDS, and so forth. Single versus double lung physiology can often be distinguished using a portable chest X-ray or point-of-care lung ultrasonography.

The importance of determining the source of a patient's shunt before intervening is that these distinct phenotypes respond differently to increases in mean airway pressure and thus tolerance to APRV. Most notably, in patients with single lung physiology, the application of a high pressure/PEEP ventilatory strategy will often lead to a paradoxic worsening of the patient's hypoxemia. This is due to a disproportionate application of pressure to the noninvolved lung leading to overdistention and worsening of the patient's shunt physiology.[17] Once the presence of single lung shunt physiology has been excluded as the source of the patient's refractory hypoxemia, APRV can be considered as an appropriate modality.

INITIAL SETTINGS AND TITRATION

APRV has 5 settings: P-high, P-low, time high (T-high), T-low, and fraction of inspired oxygen (Fio_2) (**Fig. 5**). Appropriate manipulation of these settings will optimize

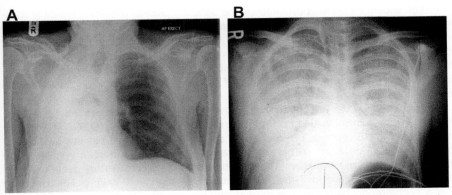

Fig. 4. (*A*) Single lung shunt physiology from complete atelectasis of the right lung causing "whiteout." (*B*) Double lung shunt physiology as manifested by opacification of both lung fields.

oxygenation, ventilation, and pulmonary mechanics for patients on APRV. It is important to keep in mind that the goal with APRV is to return patients to FRC and encourage safe spontaneous ventilation.

P-high: Pressure-high is analogous to CPAP. P-high is the maximum and sustained pressure that the ventilator will deliver during which the patient should spontaneously breathe. An appropriately set P-high will be at a pressure, which restores the patient's FRC, enabling safe, spontaneous ventilation in addition to optimal ventilation-perfusion matching. Notably, spontaneous ventilation that occurs at a higher PEEP results in more homogeneous parenchymal distension.[18]

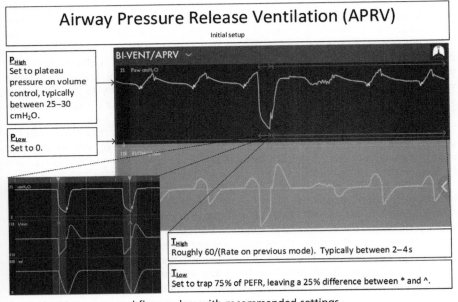

Fig. 5. APRV pressure and flow scalars with recommended settings.

P-high should be set at approximately the patient's plateau pressure, typically starting within 2 cmH$_2$O of the plateau pressure. If the patient's hypoxia worsens when initially placed on APRV, it is possible that the alveoli have distended to the point of collapsing adjacent blood vessels, preventing oxygenated blood from returning to the left heart. In this scenario, lowering P-high by 2 cmH$_2$O is reasonable. Increasing the value of P-high should be undertaken if clinicians suspect underdistension as the cause of continued hypoxemia.

T-high: The time the patient spends at the P-high between release volumes is the T-high. Typically initial values for P-high range from 25 to 35 cmH$_2$O. T-high typically ranges from 3 to 5 seconds but in cases of severe ARDS, it can be as low as 1.5 seconds. The initial goal should be to approximate the patient's minute ventilation on traditional modes of ventilation. The total time of a single respiratory cycle in APRV is the sum of T-high and T-low. Therefore, 60/(T-high + T-low) = RR. Because T-low is commonly fairly low, this formula can be simplified to 60/T-high = RR. Typically, in the ED, it is recommended to set the T-high to 2 seconds and titrate to match the patients MV requirements.

P-low: Pressure-low is the minimum pressure achieved in the respiratory cycle, typically set to 0 cmH$_2$O. It is important to note that the P-low is set to 0 cmH$_2$O to achieve the greatest pressure differential between the P-high and P-low to encourage both high peak expiratory flow rates and bulk ventilation. Although the ventilator decrements to a pressure of 0 cmH$_2$O, the patient's alveolar pressure does not. It is not the P-low that prevents derecruitment in APRV but rather the time during which the ventilator is set to stay at P-low before reengagement of the P-high. Remember, the P-low is used to achieve maximal expiratory flow rates. The T-low is the setting, which prevents derecruitment.[19] As such, even if the P-low on the ventilator is set to zero, as long as the T-low is set properly, the alveolar pressure is unlikely to decrease to zero.

T-low: T-low is arguably one of the most important settings of APRV because it controls lung volumes during bulk ventilation and prevents derecruitment and limits atelectrauma. Patients with ARDS have alveoli that collapse faster than uninjured (or less injured alveoli). A T-low that is set to allow for full exhalation would allow for alveolar collapse and, therefore, derecruitment leading to atelectrauma. In other words, T-low, as opposed to P-low, is the variable that controls end-expiratory pressure. In a patient without spontaneous ventilatory efforts, during the ventilator transition (release) from P-high to P-low, the movement of gas (exhalation), known as release volumes, allows for ventilation. There is significant heterogeneity in how clinicians set T-low.[20] Commonly, T-low is set to trap 75% of a patient's expiratory flow, "creating" a pneumatic splint.

T-low should be individually titrated to the patient's expiratory flow curve with the goal of ending T-low at approximately 75% of the PEFR (**Fig. 6**). We recommend initially starting between 0.4 and 0.5 seconds and then making smaller titrations based on the patient's individual flow curves with the goal of trapping 75%.

Returning to the clinical vignette presented at the start of the article, despite attempts to recruit on traditional modes of ventilation, a follow-up blood gas revealed no improvement in hypoxemia. Given the refractory hypoxemia with double lung-shunt physiology, the decision was made to transition the patient to APRV with the following settings. The patient's plateau pressure was found to be 28 and so a P-high of 28 was selected. P-low was set as 0. Given the patients hypercarbia despite a RR of 24, a T-high 2.0 was selected. The T-low was set to 0.4 and was measured to appropriately trap 75% of PEFR. The Fio$_2$ was maintained at 1.0 with the intent to titrate down as the lung recruited during the next few hours.

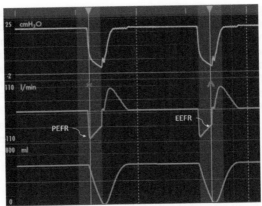

Fig. 6. APRV flow scalars demonstrating how to measure PEFR and EEFR in order to appropriately set T-low.

Once the precipitant of the hypoxic respiratory failure resolves and appropriate physiology has been restored, patients can be liberated from the ventilator. The classic strategy for weaning from APRV is known as "drop-and-stretch." "Dropping" refers to sequential decrementing of P-high and "stretching" refers to the incremental increase of T-high. Whether dropping and stretching are done in sequence or in tandem has been subject of debate. With the eventual elimination of T-low (by virtue of lengthening of T-high), the mode will no longer resemble APRV, rather, it will be CPAP.

HEMODYNAMIC CONSIDERATIONS

It is often stated that the high airway pressures used with APRV may lead to a greater degree of hemodynamic instability when compared with more traditional modes of ventilation. The observation that high airway pressures decrease preload and increase pulmonary vascular resistance gives hemodynamic consequences to APRV biological plausibility; observational data would seem to suggest it is untrue. There have been several observational studies examining patients with ARDS ventilated using APRV, in whom pulmonary artery catheters were placed. The patients were switched from traditional ventilation to APRV, and the authors observed that all hemodynamic indices improved following the initiation of APRV, including an improvement in lactate clearance and a decrease in pressor requirements.[21,22] Zhou and colleagues observed similar results in addition to a decrease in heart rate and an increase in mean arterial pressure, despite the APRV arm having significantly higher mean airway pressures.[12]

VENTILATORY CONSIDERATIONS

There is a common misconception that there is an increased rate of hypercapnia due to a decrease in the overall minute ventilation associated with the use of APRV. Never mind the more important question of whether hypercapnia is harmful in ARDS, there are numerous models demonstrating that the use of APRV promotes alveolar recruitment, improves ventilatory efficiency and increases CO_2 removal, despite a decrease in the total minute ventilation.[23,24] In a randomized control trial performed by Zhou and colleagues, the patients in the APRV group had an almost identical P_{CO_2} to the patients in the low-tidal volume group (40.8 ± 7.3 and 42.3 ± 8.6, respectively), despite using a significantly reduced minute ventilation (6.86 ± 2.06 vs 8.22 ± 2.30).

Although over time patients on APRV have lower minute ventilation requirements than patients on traditional modes of ventilation, this occurs gradually as patients improve their lung volumes. Initially, their minute ventilation requirements will be fairly close to what they were on traditional modes of ventilation. With that in mind, clinicians should endeavor to match the minute ventilation requirements previously required on standard modes of ventilation but should not be surprised if over time, these requirements decrease as patients' lung volumes begin to approximate FRC. For patients with continuous $EtCO_2$ monitoring, given the bulk of airflow occurs during T-low, the waveform will be the inverse of conventional waveforms. For patients on APRV, increasing $PETCO_2$ values may represent increasing P_{CO_2}, an increase in cardiac output, and an increasing number of alveoli now participating in ventilation.

MANAGING THE PATIENTS' RELEASE VOLUMES

Probably, the most frequent and strenuously used argument against the use of APRV is that it is often not in line with low-tidal volume ventilatory strategies and, thus, should be avoided in favor of a more traditional mode of ventilation where tidal volumes that are more precise can be obtained.

The ARMA trial published in the NEJM in 2001 examined the use of low-tidal volume ventilation in patients admitted to the ICU with ARDS. The authors found that patients randomized to a 6 cc/kg tidal volume strategy did significantly better than patients randomized to a 12 cc/kg strategy. Although this trial has a place in the tabernacle of critical care literature, the results are often misunderstood.

The ARMA trial found that patients admitted to the ICU with ARDS who were given an empiric 6 cc/kg tidal volume had a clinically significant reduction in mortality compared with patients who were given an empiric 12 cc/kg tidal volume. Or simply put, in patients with small absolute lung volumes (baby lung), a strategy that used empirically low tidal volumes was superior to a strategy that administered empirically high tidal volumes. The authors did not study whether an empiric 6 cc/kg tidal volume was optimal compared with the clinician at the bedside titrating the tidal volume to the patient's individual lung volume. Moreover, the ARMA trial was a trial examining 2 drastically different strategies of tidal volume. It did not in fact examine whether a specific mode of ventilation was optimal to any other mode of ventilation. Given the reality of ARMA, its methodology and its findings, it is nonsensical to extrapolate its findings as "proof" that a volume-cycled mode low-tidal volume strategy is superior to APRV.

A more genuine debate exists. APRV, at times, provides tidal volumes outside the safe volumes prescribed in the ARMA trial. Although release volumes may occasionally exceed 6 cc/kg, looking at tidal volumes in isolation lacks the nuanced understanding of APRV mechanics. The size of the release volume is determined by the P-high, T-low, and compliance of the patient's lung. In patients with poor compliance, due to severe ARDS, the size of the lung that is participating in ventilation is very low. In these patients, if the T-low is set to 75% of PEFR, then the release volume will also be low (often <6 cc/kg). As the patient's lung compliance improves, the release volumes will naturally increase without any change to either the P-high or the T-low. Essentially, the release volumes will be automatically tailored to the patient's individual, increasing functional lung size.

In patients with a severe reduction in lung volumes, who will truly benefit from LTV ventilation, APRV will deliver desired volumes. In patients with larger lung volumes, capable of accepting larger volumes, APRV will allow for these increased volumes. Thus, the debate should not be whether APRV is capable of delivering an LTV strategy in patients with ARDS but rather, in patients with improving compliance, is tolerating the natural increases in release volumes safe? Although the data are not definitive, studies comparing APRV to traditional modes of ventilation have failed to identify any signals of harm due to the variable tidal volumes associated with the use of APRV. In fact, most of the preclinical data demonstrate decreased strain on the individual lung units due to APRV's superior recruitment capabilities.[25–27] At least, in its limited capacity, the Zhou and colleagues trial confirmed these findings. There was no statistical difference in the rate of pneumothoraces between the 2 groups, and the point estimate noticeably favored the APRV arm (4.2% vs 10.4% *P*-value of .199).

SUMMARY

Although the precipitant of respiratory failure is being managed, MV should optimize the patient's pulmonary and hemodynamic mechanics by way of restoration of the patient's FRC. By using higher than conventional mean airway pressures with APRV, FRC is restored, and physiologic breathing can resume.

CLINICS CARE POINTS

- Airway pressure release ventilation (APRV) has 5 settings: pressure high (P-high), pressure low (P-low), time high (T-high), time low (T-low), and fraction of inspired oxygen.
- P-high: Pressure-high is analogous to continuous positive airway pressure. P-high should be set at approximately within 2 cmH_2O of the plateau pressure.
- T-high: The time the patient spends at the P-high between release volumes. It is recommended to set the T-high to 2 seconds and titrate to match the patient's mechanical ventilation requirements.
- P-low: Pressure-low is the minimum pressure achieved in the respiratory cycle, typically set to 0 cmH_2O.
- T-low: T-low is arguably one of the most important settings of APRV because it controls lung volumes during bulk ventilation and prevents derecruitment and limits atelectrauma. We recommend initially starting between 0.4 and 0.5 seconds and then making smaller titrations based on the patient's individual flow curves with the goal of trapping 75%.

DISCLOSURE

The authors have nothing to disclose.

REFERENCES

1. Mireles-Cabodevila E, Kacmarek RM. Should Airway Pressure Release Ventilation Be the Primary Mode in ARDS? Respir Care 2016;61(6):761–73.
2. Acute Respiratory Distress Syndrome Network, Brower RG, Matthay MA, et al. Ventilation with lower tidal volumes as compared with traditional tidal volumes for acute lung injury and the acute respiratory distress syndrome. N Engl J Med 2000;342(18):1301–8.
3. Writing Group for the PReVENT Investigators, Simonis FD, Serpa Neto A, et al. Effect of a Low vs Intermediate Tidal Volume Strategy on Ventilator-Free Days in Intensive Care Unit Patients Without ARDS: A Randomized Clinical Trial. JAMA 2018;320(18):1872–80.
4. Máca J, Jor O, Holub M, et al. Past and Present ARDS Mortality Rates: A Systematic Review. Respir Care 2017;62(1):113–22.

5. Guérin C, Reignier J, Richard J-C, et al. Prone positioning in severe acute respiratory distress syndrome. N Engl J Med 2013;368(23):2159–68.
6. Gattinoni L, Pesenti A. The concept of "baby lung. Intensive Care Med 2005; 31(6):776–84.
7. Katira BH. Ventilator-Induced Lung Injury: Classic and Novel Concepts. Respir Care 2019;64(6):629–37.
8. Slutsky AS, Ranieri VM. Ventilator-induced lung injury. N Engl J Med 2013; 369(22):2126–36.
9. Williams EC, Motta-Ribeiro GC, Vidal Melo MF. Driving Pressure and Transpulmonary Pressure: How Do We Guide Safe Mechanical Ventilation? Anesthesiology 2019;131(1):155–63.
10. West JB. Respiratory physiology: the essentials. Philidelphia: Lippincott Williams & Wilkins; 2008.
11. Jain SV, Kollisch-Singule M, Sadowitz B, et al. The 30-year evolution of airway pressure release ventilation (APRV). Intensive Care Med Exp 2016;4(1):11.
12. Zhou Y, Jin X, Lv Y, et al. Early application of airway pressure release ventilation may reduce the duration of mechanical ventilation in acute respiratory distress syndrome. Intensive Care Med 2017;43(11):1648–59.
13. Lim J, Litton E. Airway Pressure Release Ventilation in Adult Patients With Acute Hypoxemic Respiratory Failure: A Systematic Review and Meta-Analysis. Crit Care Med 2019;47(12):1794–9.
14. Andrews PL, Shiber JR, Jaruga-Killeen E, et al. Early application of airway pressure release iventilation may reduce mortality in high-risk trauma patients: a systematic review of observational trauma ARDS literature. J Trauma Acute Care Surg 2013;75(4):635–41.
15. Ge H, Lin L, Xu Y, et al. Airway Pressure Release Ventilation Mode Improves Circulatory and Respiratory Function in Patients After Cardiopulmonary Bypass, a Randomized Trial. Front Physiol 2021;12:684927.
16. Kallet RH, Burns G, Zhuo H, et al. Severity of Hypoxemia and Other Factors That Influence the Response to Aerosolized Prostacyclin in ARDS. Respir Care 2017; 62(8):1014–22.
17. Çoruh B, Luks AM. Positive end-expiratory pressure. When more may not be better. Ann Am Thorac Soc 2014;11(8):1327–31.
18. Yoshida T, Grieco DL, Brochard L, et al. Patient self-inflicted lung injury and positive end-expiratory pressure for safe spontaneous breathing. Curr Opin Crit Care 2020;26(1):59–65.
19. Coppola S, Caccioppola A, Froio S, et al. Dynamic hyperinflation and intrinsic positive end-expiratory pressure in ARDS patients. Crit Care 2019;23(1):375.
20. Miller AG, Gentile MA, Davies JD, et al. Clinical Management Strategies for Airway Pressure Release Ventilation: A Survey of Clinical Practice. Respir Care 2017;62(10):1264–8.
21. Taha A, Shafie A, Mostafa M, et al. Airway pressure release ventilation restores hemodynamic stability in patients with cardiogenic shock: initial experience in cardiac intensive care. Crit Care 2014;18(1):1–182.
22. Kaplan LJ, Bailey H, Formosa V. Airway pressure release ventilation increases cardiac performance in patients with acute lung injury/adult respiratory distress syndrome. Crit Care 2001;5(4):221–6.
23. Knelson JH, Howatt WF, DeMuth GR. Effect of respiratory pattern on alveolar gas exchange. J Appl Physiol 1970;29(3):328–31.
24. Fuleihan SF, Wilson RS, Pontoppidan H. Effect of mechanical ventilation with end-inspiratory pause on blood-gas exchange. Anesth Analg 1976;55(1):122–30.

25. Kollisch-Singule M, Emr B, Smith B, et al. Mechanical breath profile of airway pressure release ventilation: the effect on alveolar recruitment and microstrain in acute lung injury. JAMA Surg 2014;149(11):1138–45.
26. Kollisch-Singule M, Emr B, Smith B, et al. Airway pressure release ventilation reduces conducting airway micro-strain in lung injury. J Am Coll Surg 2014;219(5): 968–76.
27. Kollisch-Singule M, Jain S, Andrews P, et al. Effect of Airway Pressure Release Ventilation on Dynamic Alveolar Heterogeneity. JAMA Surg 2016;151(1):64–72.

Infectious Pulmonary Diseases

Rachel Rafeq, PharmD[a],*, Lauren A. Igneri, PharmD, BCPS, BCCCP[b,1]

KEYWORDS

- Community-acquired pneumonia • Hospital-acquired pneumonia
- Ventilator-associated pneumonia • Antimicrobial stewardship • Allergies
- Cross-sensitivity • Procalcitonin • MRSA nasal screening

KEY POINTS

- Community-acquired pneumonia is most commonly caused by *Streptococcus pneumoniae* and requires various antimicrobial therapy depending on patient disposition and severity of disease.
- Patients with hospital-acquired and ventilator-associated pneumonia are at risk for multidrug-resistant pathogens, especially following exposure to intravenous antibiotics within the last 90 days.
- Immunocompromised populations may require broader spectrum antimicrobial therapy to accommodate additional organisms not typically seen in non-immunocompromised populations.
- Although guidelines serve as an important source for appropriate treatment of pneumonia, a shift in emphasizing individualized approaches to antibiotic therapy is needed to improve patient outcomes.

INTRODUCTION

Pneumonia is a lower respiratory tract infection caused by the inability to clear pathogens from the lower airway and alveoli. Cytokines and local inflammatory markers are released, causing further damage to the lungs through an inflammatory cascade leading to an accumulation of white blood cells and fluid congestion, leading to pus in the parenchyma. The Infectious Diseases Society of America (IDSA) defines pneumonia as the presence of new lung infiltrate with other clinical evidence supporting infection,

No commercial or financial conflicts of interest or any funding sources to disclose.

Statement of authorship – both authors contributed equally to this article.

[a] Emergency Medicine, Department of Pharmacy, Cooper University Healthcare, 1 Cooper Plaza, Camden, NJ 08103, USA; [b] Critical Care, Department of Pharmacy, Cooper University Healthcare, 1 Cooper Plaza, Camden, NJ 08103, USA

[1] Author contributed equally to the publication of this article

* Corresponding author.

E-mail address: rafeq-rachel@cooperhealth.edu

including new fever, purulent sputum, leukocytosis, and decline in oxygenation. Importantly, lower respiratory infections remain the deadliest communicable disease. Ranking as the fourth leading cause of death worldwide, 2.6 million lives were claimed from pneumonia in 2019.

COMMUNITY-ACQUIRED PNEUMONIA

Community-acquired pneumonia (CAP) is a leading cause of hospitalization and death in the United States with more than 1.5 million Americans hospitalized annually.[1] It accounts for 4.5 million outpatient and emergency department visits annually. Up to 30% of mortality among intensive care unit (ICU) patients are related to pneumonia, with *S pneumoniae* remaining the most common bacterial pathogen implicated in CAP despite vaccine availability.[2] The understanding of microbiologic studies and inflammatory markers, such as procalcitonin (PCT), can be used to guide management. The American Thoracic Society (ATS) and the IDSA provide antibiotic recommendations, which will vary depending on whether outpatient or inpatient management is required.

Etiology

Several bacterial pathogens and some viral and fungal pathogens are implicated in the cause of CAP including:[3]

Bacterial Pathogen	Characteristics
Streptococcus pneumonia	• Aerobic, gram-positive diplococcus. • The most common cause of CAP; however, the incidence has decreased over the years with the widespread use of pneumococcal vaccine.
Haemophilus influenza	• Aerobic gram-negative coccobacillus. • Spread person to person via airborne droplets or through direct contact with respiratory secretions of an infected or colonized individual.
Legionella pneumophila	• Atypical pathogen • Gram-negative bacilli, classified as an atypical pneumonia. • Implicated in <4% of all CAP cases.
Mycoplasma pneumonia	• Atypical pathogen • Unlike other bacteria, it does not contain a cell wall rendering beta-lactam antimicrobial ineffective. • Unable to be gram stained due to the lack of cell wall.
Chlamydia pneumonia	• Atypical pathogen • Obligate intracellular gram-negative bacteria.
Moraxella catarrhalis	• Gram-negative diplococcus that commonly produces beta-lactamase, rendering it mostly resistant to amoxicillin. • Most frequently found as part of normal flora in infants and children but decreases in adults.
Pseudomonas aeruginosa	• Implicated in up to 8.3% of severe CAP requiring ICU admissions. • Pseudomonal infection is associated with poorer clinical outcomes and multidrug resistance.

- Viruses
  - CAP pathogens include coronaviruses (in 2020, primarily SARS-CoV-2), influenza A, RSV, parainfluenzea, adenovirus, human metapneumovirus, and rhinovirus.
  - The Center for Disease report of 2300 adults hospitalized with CAP showed the most common identified pathogens were rhinovirus (9%), influenza (6%), and *S pneumoniae* (5%). No pathogens were identified in 62% of cases.

- Pathogens to be considered in special circumstances (eg, immunocompromised)
  - *Mycobacterium tuberculosis*
  - *Nocardia* spp.
  - *Pneumocystis jirovecii*
  - *Aspergillus spp.*
  - *Mucorales spp.*
  - *Varicella-zoster virus*
  - *Cytomegalovirus*
  - Group A *Streptococcus*
  - *Neisseria meningitidis*
  - Anaerobes (aspiration pneumonia)

Prognosis Assessment Tools

Clinical comorbidities and social habits (eg, smoking) may worsen or increase the risk of CAP. The pneumonia severity index (PSI) and CURB-65 are assessment tools used to predict 30-day mortality in immunocompetent patients (**Tables 1** and **2**).[4] PSI is recommended over CURB-65 because it has a higher discriminative power in predicting mortality .[5]

Diagnostic Strategies

Microbiologic studies are integral to guiding antimicrobial treatment and vary depending on whether outpatient or inpatient management is required. In the outpatient setting, pretreatment sputum gram stain, the culture of the lower respiratory secretions, and blood cultures are not recommended.[5] However, these studies are crucial in hospital patients, particularly in patients being managed for severe CAP or the patients who are empirically treated for methicillin-resistant *Staphylococcus aureus* (MRSA) or *Pseudomonas aeruginosa*. In addition, these tests should be performed for all patients previously infected with MRSA or *Pseudomonas* spp., or who were hospitalized and received intravenous antibiotics in the last 90 days. In patients with severe CAP, urine *Legionella* and pneumococcal antigen testing are recommended.[5]

The 2019 CAP guidelines address the use of PCT and corticosteroids, which differs from the prior 2007 guideline. PCT, regardless of level, is not recommended to determine the need for empiric antibiotic initiation. Instead, clinical criteria and radiographically confirmed infiltrate should guide the administration of antimicrobials. Although corticosteroids also are not recommended for routine use, they may be considered in patients with septic shock (**Table 3**).[5]

Therapeutic Options

Antimicrobial treatment is initiated on an empiric basis and in hospitalized patients may be streamlined once the causative organism is identified (**Tables 4** and **5**).

The etiology of disease is important for several reasons. As empiric therapy tends to be broad to cover a wide range of possible pathogens, the culture results will allow providers to narrow therapy and determine resistance if applicable.

Risk factors for MRSA or *P aeruginosa*:[5]

- Prior respiratory isolation of MRSA or *P aeruginosa*
- Recent hospitalization plus receipt of parenteral antibiotics in the last 90 days

Table 1
Pneumonia severity index

Patient Characteristics			Points Assigned
Demographic Factors			
Age			1 point per year
Men			Age (y)
Women			Age (y) − 10
Nursing home resident			+ 10
Comorbid Illnesses			
Neoplastic disease			+30
Liver disease			+20
Congestive heart disease			+10
Cerebrovascular disease			+10
Renal disease			+10
Physical examination findings			
Altered mental status			+ 20
Respiratory rate ≥ 30 breaths/min			+ 20
Systolic blood pressure <90 mmHg			+ 20
Temperature <30° or ≥40° C			+ 15
Pulse ≥125 beats/min			+ 10
Laboratory findings			
PH <7.35			+30
blood *urea* nitrogen >10.7 mmol/L			+20
Sodium <130 meq/L			+20
Glucose >13.9 mmol/L			+10
Hematocrit <30%			+10
$PO_2 < 60$ mmHg (or $SaO_2 < 90\%$)			+10
Pleural effusion			+10

Risk Class	Points Total	Mortality Rate	Patient Care Location
I	<51	0.1%	Outpatient
II	51–70	0.6%	Outpatient
III	71–90	2.8%	Observation unit with reevaluation if possible
IV	91–130	8.2%	Inpatient
V	>130	29.2%	Inpatient, likely ICU

Aspiration Pneumonia

In the new 2019 guidelines, the IDSA/ATS suggest not routinely adding anaerobic coverage for suspected aspiration pneumonia unless there is suspicion of or known lung empyema or abscess. Many patients with aspiration pneumonia are found to have self-limiting symptoms that resolve in 24 to 48 hours and only require supportive care without the need for antibiotics. Avoidance of unnecessary antimicrobial therapy has become paramount in light of the growing body of evidence for increased *Clostridioides difficile* infection and multidrug-resistant (MDR) pathogens associated with broad-spectrum antimicrobials (eg, cefepime, ceftriaxone, carbapenems, fluoroquinolones, clindamycin, and so forth).[5]

Table 2
CURB-65 criteria

Characteristics	Points Total
Confusion	1
Increased blood urea nitrogen >20 mg/dL	1
Respiratory rate ≥30 breaths/min	1
Blood pressure (systolic BP <90 mmHg or diastolic ≤60 mmHg)	1
Age >65 y	1

Total Score	Recommendation
0–1	Low risk; outpatient treatment
2	Moderately severe; short inpatient hospitalization or closely supervised outpatient treatment
3–5	Severe pneumonia; hospitalization required; consider intensive care unit admission

Antimicrobial Dosing

Although the CAP guidelines provide clear dosing recommendations for some treatment options, dosing ranges are provided for severe infection treatment options to allow clinicians selection of an optimal dose based on patient-specific characteristics. A systematic review and meta-analysis by Telles and colleagues evaluated the efficacy of ceftriaxone 1 g versus 2 g daily for the treatment of CAP based on data pooled from 24 randomized controlled trials. Of note, trials including critically ill patients were excluded: 12 studies evaluated ceftriaxone 1 g and 12 studies evaluated ceftriaxone 2 g. Comparator regimens show similar efficacy ceftriaxone 1 g daily dosing [OR 1.03 (95% CI [0.88–1.20])], and dosages higher than ceftriaxone 1 g daily did not result in improved clinical outcomes for CAP (OR 1.02, 95% CI [0.91–1.14]).[6]

Hasegawa and colleagues supported these findings in their evaluation of ceftriaxone 1-g versus 2-g daily dosing. A similar rate of clinical cure was seen with ceftriaxone 1 g (94.6%) versus 2 g (93.1%), risk difference 1.5% (95% CI 3.1–6.0, $P = .009$ for non-inferiority). These studies prove that ceftriaxone 1 g daily is as safe and effective as other CAP regimens, including higher ceftriaxone dosing.[7] This is important as clinicians look to reduce antimicrobial resistance by minimizing excessive antimicrobial exposure.

Table 3
Severe community-acquired pneumonia criteria[5]

Severe CAP Is Defined as Having Three or More Minor Criteria OR One Major Criteria	
Minor criteria	• Confusion/disorientation • Hypotension requiring aggressive fluid resuscitation • Hypothermia (core temperature <36°C) • Leukopenia from infection along (ie, not related to chemotherapy) defined as white blood cell count <4000 cells/μL • Multilobar infiltrates • PaO_2/FiO_2 ratio ≤250 • Respiratory rate ≥30 breaths/min • Uremia (blood urea nitrogen level ≥20 mg/dL)
Major criteria	• Respiratory failure requiring mechanical ventilation • Septic shock with the need for vasopressors

Table 4
Outpatient community-acquired pneumonia therapeutic options[5]

Patient Characteristics	Antimicrobial Therapy of Choice
No comorbidities or risk factors for MRSA or *P aeruginosa*	• Amoxicillin 1 g oral three times daily OR • Doxycycline 100 mg oral twice daily OR • Azithromycin[a] 500 mg oral on day 1, azithromycin, 250 mg oral on days 2–4 • Clarithromycin[a] 500 mg oral twice daily or clarithromycin ER 1000 mg oral daily
With comorbidities[b]	• Combination therapy with: • Amoxicillin/clavulanate 500 mg/125 mg three times oral daily, amoxicillin/clavulanate 875 mg/125 mg oral twice daily, amoxicillin/clavulanate 2000 mg/125 mg oral twice daily, cefpodoxime 200 mg oral twice daily, or cefuroxime 500 mg oral twice daily AND Azithromycin, 500 mg oral on the first day then 250 mg oral daily, clarithromycin 500 mg oral twice daily, clarithromycin ER 1000 mg oral daily, or doxycycline 100 mg oral twice daily • Monotherapy with respiratory fluoroquinolone levofloxacin 750 mg oral daily, moxifloxacin 400 mg oral daily, or gemifloxacin 320 mg oral daily

[a] Use macrolides only if local pneumococcal resistance is less than 25%.
[b] Chronic heart, liver, lung or renal disease, diabetes mellitus, alcoholism, malignancy, or asplenia.

Treatment Duration

Treatment duration varies based on the resolution of vital sign abnormalities, ability to eat, and normal mentation. IDSA recommends no less than 5 days of therapy in uncomplicated outpatient CAP, and several meta-analysis studies have demonstrated successful efficacy with 5 to 7 day treatment durations.[5,8–10] Inpatient CAP treatment should also be not less than 5 days unless MRSA or *P aeruginosa* is involved, then it is not less than 7 days.

In patients with complicated CAP, such as those with concurrent meningitis or endocarditis, 5 to 7 days of treatment is not sufficient, and longer durations are warranted.[5] PCT may be a useful biomarker to help guide treatment duration and is discussed further in the Antimicrobial Stewardship section.

HOSPITAL-ACQUIRED PNEUMONIA

The IDSA, the ATS, and international guidelines define hospital-acquired pneumonia (HAP) as a nosocomial infection of the lung parenchyma not present at the time of hospital admission that develops in patients after 48 hours of hospitalization. A subtype of HAP is ventilator-associated pneumonia (VAP), occurring in patients who have required mechanical ventilation for at least 48 hours.[11,12] Health care-associated pneumonia (HCAP) had previously been included in the HAP and VAP guidelines, but it was removed in the most recent update as new literature demonstrates that patients with HCAP are not at high risk for MDR pathogens as previously thought and are probably better categorized within the CAP guidelines.[11]

Diagnostic Strategies

In nosocomial pneumonia, microbiological studies should be performed before initiation of antimicrobial therapy to guide definitive therapy.

Noninvasive, qualitative, or semiquantitative cultures (eg, spontaneous expectoration, sputum inductions, nasotracheal suctioning, and endotracheal aspiration) are preferred over invasive, quantitative sampling strategies (eg, bronchial-alveolar lavage, protected specimen brush, and blind bronchial sampling) as no statistically significant difference in mortality rates were found between quantitative and qualitative cultures (RR 0.91; 95% CI 0.75–1.11).[13] No difference in other clinical outcomes, including duration of mechanical ventilation, ICU length of stay, and antibiotic change, were seen with the two sampling strategies.[13] In addition, noninvasive sampling can be performed rapidly and avoid delays in the initiation of effective antimicrobial therapy.[11] Blood cultures should be obtained for patients with suspected HAP/VAP as they may provide insight into the severity of illness and direct antimicrobial initiation and ultimately play a role in determining appropriate definitive therapy.

In general, clinical criteria for pneumonia should guide the initiation of empiric antimicrobial therapy in HAP/VAP. Although biomarkers such as PCT, c-reactive protein, or bronchial alveolar fluid soluble triggering receptor expressed on myeloid cells (sTREM-1) have been studied for the initiation of antimicrobial therapy in HAP/VAP, none have been associated with acceptable sensitivity or specificity for the diagnosis of HAP/VAP compared with using clinical criteria alone.[11]

Therapeutic Options

Although prior guidelines differentiated empiric treatment for nosocomial pneumonia based on the bacteriology of disease onset, early (within 4 days) versus late (5 days or more), recent literature indicates that patients with the early-onset disease may still be at risk for MDR pathogens.[12] Therefore, risk stratification for MDR organisms should not be based solely on disease onset. Prior intravenous antibiotic use within the last 90 days is the major risk factor for the development of MDR (eg, MRSA, *Pseudomonas* spp., and so forth), VAP (OR 12.3; 95% CI 6.48–23.35), and HAP (OR 5.17; 95% CI 2.11–12.67).[11] In addition, patients with VAP may be at increased risk of MDR pathogens when infection occurs on hospital day 5 or later or is complicated by septic shock, acute respiratory distress syndrome (ARDS), or need for acute renal replacement therapy.[11]

Empiric antimicrobial therapy selections for HAP and VAP should be stratified based on patient risk factors for MDR pathogens, as outlined in **Tables 6** and **7**. Antipseudomonal beta-lactam therapy is the cornerstone of nosocomial pneumonia treatment. Empiric, dual antipseudomonal coverage from different antibiotic classes is indicated in VAP when the patient has a risk factor for MDR pathogen, greater than 10% of gram-negative isolates are resistant to the antimicrobial being considered for monotherapy or local ICU susceptibilities are unavailable, and in HAP when there is a risk for MDR pathogen, need for mechanical ventilation, or presence of shock.[11] However, dual antipseudomonal therapy is controversial, and ultimately local sensitivities should be taken into consideration when determining empiric therapy. Intensivists should collaborate with antimicrobial stewardship (AMS) to develop local treatment pathways that are based on the national guidelines but are tailored to local data.[14]

Anti-MRSA antimicrobials are indicated for patients with HAP or VAP when there is a risk factor for MDR organisms or if an infection develops in hospital wards whereby greater than 10% to 20% of *Staphylococcus aureus* are methicillin-resistant. Otherwise, empiric treatment for HAP or VAP should target methicillin-sensitive *S aureus*.[11]

Clinical Considerations with Antimicrobial Selection and Dosing

Patient-specific factors including allergy history, organ function, and concomitant medications should be evaluated when selecting empiric antimicrobial regimens.

Table 5
Inpatient community-acquired pneumonia therapeutic options[5]

	NO Risk for *P aeruginosa* or MRSA
Non-severe	Combination therapy with ampicillin–sulbactam 1.5–3 g IV every 6 h, cefotaxime 1–2 g IV every 8 h, ceftriaxone 1–2 g IV daily, or ceftaroline 600 mg IV every 12 h Plus Azithromycin 500 mg oral or IV daily or clarithromycin 500 mg oral twice daily OR monotherapy with levofloxacin 750 mg oral or IV daily or moxifloxacin 400 mg oral or IV daily
Severe	Combination therapy with ampicillin–sulbactam 1.5–3 g IV every 6 h, cefotaxime 1–2 g IV every 8 h, ceftriaxone 1–2 g IV daily, or ceftaroline 600 mg IV every 12 h Plus Azithromycin 500 mg oral or IV daily or clarithromycin 500 mg oral twice daily OR Levofloxacin 750 mg oral or IV daily or moxifloxacin 400 mg oral or IV daily
	WITH Risk Factors for *P aeruginosa* or MRSA
MRSA	If prior respiratory isolation of MRSA, IV antibiotics within the last 90 d, suspected necrotizing pneumonia or empyema regardless of non-severe or severe CAP • MRSA coverage: Vancomycin 15 mg/kg IV every 12 h (adjusted with TDM) or linezolid IV 600 mg every 12 h • Obtain cultures/nasal MRSA PCR to allow for de-escalation or confirmation of the need to continue therapy
P aeruginosa	If prior respiratory isolation of *P aeruginosa*, hospitalization within the last 90 d and receipt of intravenous antibiotics within the last 90 d regardless of non-severe or severe CAP • Piperacillin–tazobactam 4.5 g IV every 6 h, cefepime 2 g IV every 8 h, ceftazidime 2 g IV every 8 h, imipenem 500 mg IV every 6 h, meropenem 1 g IV every 8 h, or aztreonam 2 g IV every 8 h • Obtain cultures to allow for de-escalation or confirmation of the need to continue therapy

Historically, piperacillin–tazobactam with vancomycin was recommended for empiric HAP/VAP treatment. However, a recent literature shows the odds of acute kidney injury with vancomycin plus piperacillin–tazobactam are significantly increased compared with vancomycin monotherapy (OR 3.40; 95% CI 2.57–4.50), vancomycin plus cefepime or carbapenem therapy (OR 2.68; 95% CI 1.83–3.91), or piperacillin-tazobactam monotherapy (OR 2.70; 95% CI 1.97–3.69).[15] Therefore, the use of cefepime in place of piperacillin–tazobactam may be preferable to avoid potential nephrotoxicity complications.

Linezolid may increase the risk of serotonin syndrome when given with serotonergic medications (eg, selective serotonin reuptake inhibitors, serotonin–norepinephrine reuptake inhibitors, serotonin receptor agonists, tricyclic antidepressants, monoamine oxidase inhibitors, and opioid medications.)[11] If linezolid is chosen as either empiric or definitive therapy for HAP/VAP, careful screening for other serotonergic medications is needed. Temporary cessation of concurrent serotonergic medications may be needed if linezolid remains the preferred anti-MRSA therapy.

Pharmacokinetic (PK)-optimized/pharmacodynamic (PD)-optimized antimicrobial dosing should be used when treating serious infections. As antipseudomonal beta-

Table 6
Empiric antimicrobial therapy for hospital-acquired pneumonia[11]

Patient Characteristics	Antimicrobial Therapy Choices	
High risk of mortality[a] or received IV antimicrobials in the past 90 d	Select two of the following, avoid double beta-lactam therapy or same drug class: • Piperacillin–tazobactam 4.5 g IV every 6 h • Cefepime or ceftazidime 2 g IV every 8 h • Levofloxacin, 750 mg IV daily or ciprofloxacin 400 mg IV every 8 h • Imipenem 500 mg IV every 6 h or meropenem 1 g IV every 8 h • Amikacin 15–20 mg/kg IV daily • Gentamicin or tobramycin 5–7 mg/kg IV daily • Aztreonam 2 g IV every 8 h	Plus anti-MRSA therapy: • Vancomycin, 25–30 mg/kg IV once followed by 15 mg/kg IV every 8–12 h with TDM targeting through 15–20 mg/mL, or • Linezolid 600 mg IV every 12 h
Not high risk of mortality, but MRSA risk factor(s) present[b]	Select two of the following, avoid double beta-lactam therapy or same drug class: • Piperacillin–tazobactam 4.5 g IV every 6 h • Cefepime or ceftazidime, 2 g IV every 8 h • Levofloxacin 750 mg IV daily or ciprofloxacin 400 mg IV every 8 h • Imipenem 500 mg IV every 6 h or meropenem 1 g IV every 8 h • Aztreonam 2 g IV every 8 h	Plus anti-MRSA therapy: • Vancomycin 25–30 mg/kg IV once followed by 15 mg/kg IV every 8–12 h with TDM targeting through 15–20 mg/mL or • Linezolid 600 mg IV every 12 h
Not high risk of mortality and no MRSA risk factor(s) present[b]	Select one of the following: • Piperacillin–tazobactam 4.5 g IV every 6 h • Cefepime or ceftazidime 2 g IV every 8 h • Levofloxacin 750 mg IV daily or • Imipenem 500 mg IV every 6 h • Meropenem 1 g IV every 8 h	

[a] High risk for mortality: requiring ventilatory support or presence of septic shock.
[b] MRSA risk factors: prior intravenous antibiotic use within the last 90 d, hospital wards with greater than 10% to 20% MRSA isolates.

lactam therapy is the backbone of nosocomial pneumonia treatment, the time-free drug concentrations are above the minimum inhibitory concentration (fT > MIC) must be enhanced. Critically ill patients with altered hemodynamics and organ function may benefit from the use of prolonged or continuous infusion dosing strategies and the emerging practice of beta-lactam TDM to ensure PK/PD goals are

Table 7
Empiric antibiotic therapy for ventilator-associated pneumonia[11]

Patient Characteristics	Antimicrobial Therapy Choices	
• Received IV antimicrobials in the past 90 d • Septic shock at onset of VAP • ARDS preceding VAP • Acute renal replacement therapy preceding VAP • VAP onset hospital day 5 or later	Select one agent from each category: β-lactams • Piperacillin–tazobactam 4.5 g IV every 6 h • Cefepime or ceftazidime 2 g IV every 8 h • Imipenem 500 mg IV every 6 h or meropenem 1 g IV every 8 h • Aztreonam 2 g IV every 8 h Non-β-lactams • Levofloxacin 750 mg IV daily or ciprofloxacin 400 mg IV every 8 h • Amikacin 15–20 mg/kg IV daily • Gentamicin or tobramycin 5–7 mg/kg IV daily • Colistin 5 mg/kg IV loading dose followed by maintenance dose (2.5 mg*CrCl + 30) IV every 12 h or polymyxin B 2.5–3.0 mg/kg/d divided twice daily	Plus anti-MRSA therapy: • Vancomycin 25–30 mg/kg IV once followed by 15 mg/kg IV every 8–12 h with TDM targeting through 15–20 mg/mL or • Linezolid 600 mg IV every 12 h

met.[11,14,16] In addition, vancomycin dosing and monitoring strategies have shifted to targeting an area under the curve to a MIC ratio of ≥ 400.[17] Future nosocomial pneumonia guidelines should be updated to reflect recommended vancomycin PD targets.

Definitive Therapy

Culture data revealing antimicrobial susceptibility testing should guide definitive antimicrobial therapy. In general, empiric regimens should be de-escalated to the most narrow spectrum agent covering the pathogen to avoid complications, such as *Clostridioides difficile* infection.[14] However, in cases whereby pathogens express expanded-spectrum beta-lactamases or carbapenem resistance, antimicrobial therapy should be targeted to treat these organisms.[11] Patients with pneumonia secondary to MDR gram-negative bacilli only sensitive to aminoglycosides or colistin may benefit from the initiation of inhaled antimicrobial therapy in addition to IV systemic therapy.[11]

Treatment Duration

Historically, HAP/VAP were treated for long durations up to 2 weeks, but updated evidence demonstrates that 7 days of therapy is suitable for most patients.[11] One pivotal clinical trial showed that 8 days of VAP treatment was non-inferior to 15 days in that there was no significant difference in mortality (18.8% vs 17.2%, difference 1.6%, 90% CI -3.7%–6.9%) or recurrent infection (28.9% vs 26.0%, difference 2.9%, 90% CI -3.2%–9.1%), but increased mean ± SD antimicrobial-free days in the 8 days group (13.1 ± 7.4 vs 8.7 ± 5.2, P<.001).[18] However, a subgroup of patients with non-lactose fermenting pathogens (eg, P aeruginosa) had a higher rate of recurrent infections, which was confirmed in one meta-analysis.[18,19] Updated meta-analyses of HAP/VAP treatment duration did not show a significant difference in recurrent infections with shorter courses regardless of the causative pathogen.[11,20]

Ultimately, clinical criteria should guide HAP/VAP resolution and antimicrobial discontinuation. Select populations may require an individualized duration of treatment, including those with severe immunocompromised state, initially treated with inappropriate antibiotic therapy or highly resistant pathogens, including P aeruginosa or carbapenem-resistant Enterobacteriaceae or Acinetobacter spp.[12]

IMMUNOCOMPROMISED POPULATIONS

Immunocompromised populations are at increased risk of pneumonia from both common pathogens and avirulent or opportunistic organisms.[21] Immunocompromised conditions include, but are not limited to receipt of cancer chemotherapy, solid organ transplantation, hematopoietic stem cell transplantation, HIV infection with a CD4 T-lymphocyte count less than 200 cells/microliter or percentage less than 14%, or receipt of corticosteroid therapy with a dose greater than 20 mg prednisone or equivalent daily for greater than 14 days or a cumulative dose greater than 600 mg of prednisone.[21]

Although immunocompromised patients may develop an infection from the typical CAP respiratory pathogens, they are also at risk for infection due to Enterobacteriaceae (including extended-spectrum beta-lactamase and carbapenemase-producing organisms), mycobacteria (eg, Mycobacterium tuberculosis), viruses (eg, Cytomegalovirus), fungi (eg, Pneumocystis jirovecii), and parasites (eg, Toxoplasma gondii).[21] Broad-spectrum therapy targeting beyond core respiratory pathogens should be used empirically when risk factors for MDR or opportunistic pathogens exist, and the delay in appropriate therapy will place the patient at increased risk of mortality.

Immunocompromised patients should be managed on a case-by-case basis to ensure pathogen-directed therapy is initiated, as shown **Table 8**.[21] Although a discussion on newer beta-lactam/beta-lactamase inhibitor combinations (eg, ceftolozane/tazobactam, imipenem/relabactam, meropenem/vaborbactam, and so forth) for the treatment of MDR gram-negative bacilli is beyond the scope of this review, there may be a role for these agents in the place of systemic aminoglycoside or colistin when treating highly resistant pathogens (eg, extended-spectrum beta-lactamase producing Enterobacteriaceae and carbapenem-resistant Enterobacteriaceae) under the direction of an infectious disease specialist.

ANTIMICROBIAL STEWARDSHIP INITIATIVES
Beta-Lactam Allergies

Beta-lactam intolerance (eg, gastrointestinal upset) is often misconstrued as a true allergic reaction and inappropriately documented in the patient chart. This may potentially result in an inferior or unnecessarily broad-spectrum antibiotic prescribing. Although beta-lactam antibiotics are the most common cause of drug-induced delayed rashes, including maculopapular, they infrequently cause true IgE-mediated reactions. Anaphylaxis is rare for penicillin: 0.001% for the parenteral route of administration and 0.0005% for the oral route of administration.[22]

Beta-lactam allergies documented in the medical record should be carefully reviewed to determine if a true allergy exists or whether the allergy is, in fact, a mislabel. Clarification of mislabeled allergies should be made in the medical record to alert other providers of intolerances that may not preclude the use of first-line treatment. When a true allergy exists, cross-reactivity between beta-lactam antibiotics must be carefully evaluated to avoid inappropriate exclusion of the entire class in the management of pneumonia.

Cross-reactivity between beta-lactams depends on the R1 side chain of the chemical structure. Therefore, an antibiotic with the same R1 side chain as the drug allergy should not be selected, and an alternative agent should be considered. For example, cephalexin and cefaclor have an identical side chain to amoxicillin.[22]

First generation cephalosporins have a higher cross-reactivity risk with penicillins compared to fourth generation cephalosporins due to similarities in the R1 side chain.[23] The cross-reactivity between penicillins and carbapenems, as well as carbapenems and cephalosporins, is less than 1%.[23] Monobactams do not cross-react with penicillins or carbapenems and could serve as a safe alternative agent in patients with a true risk of IgE reaction. If the R1 side chains are the same or similar, then clinical judgment should be used to determine if the reaction should be challenged.

Procalcitonin

PCT is a precursor hormone of calcitonin that is upregulated by cytokines released in response to bacterial infections. With a half-life of 25 to 30 hours, a rapid rise in PCT levels is seen within 6 to 12 hours of bacterial insult which decline as the infection resolves. Although PCT was first approved by the FDA in 2005 as a diagnostic aid for sepsis, it has proven useful as a tool for antimicrobial de-escalation.[24]

Numerous randomized studies have examined whether PCT-based algorithms can assist clinicians in deciding whether to start or stop antimicrobial therapy without adversely impacting patients through delayed antimicrobial therapy or inadequate treatment courses.[24] Efficacy has been demonstrated in adult patients with suspected respiratory infections. Improving antibiotic use in these scenarios carries the potential for important clinical benefit as respiratory infections are the most common indication for antibiotics in hospitalized patients, and antibiotic use is most prevalent in the ICU.

A systematic review and meta-analysis by Lam *and colleagues* evaluated PCT-guided antibiotic cessation (using PCT drop of 50%–90% from baseline with an absolute value <0.5–1 mcg/L) compared with standard of care in adult critically ill patients

Table 8
Pathogen-directed therapy for immunocompromised patients[21]

Pathogen	Empiric Treatment
P jirovecci	Trimethoprim–sulfamethoxazole 15–20 mg/kg/d divided every 6–8 h
Nocardia spp.	Trimethoprim–sulfamethoxazole 15–20 mg/kg/d divided every 6–8 h
Aspergillus spp.	Preferred: Liposomal amphotericin, 5–7.5 mg/kg/d Alternative: Isavuconazole, 200 mg every 8 h (initial dosing)
Mucorales spp.	Preferred: Liposomal amphotericin 5–7.5 mg/kg/d Alternative: Isavuconazole 200 mg every 8 h (initial dosing)
Varicella-zoster virus	Acyclovir 10–15 mg/kg IV every 8 h
Cytomegalovirus	Ganciclovir 5 mg/kg IV every 12 h

Table 9	
Common causes of false-positive and false-negative procalcitonin results	
False-Positive	**False-Negative**
Burns	Abscesses
Circulatory shock	Empyema
Inhalation injury	Mediastinitis
Pancreatitis	
Severe trauma	
Surgery	

was associated with a decrease in 30-day mortality, RR 0.87 (95% CI 0.77–0.98, P = .02). However, there was no decrease in short-term mortality when PCT was used for either initiation or initiation and cessation of antibiotics.[25] In addition, they demonstrated that PCT-guided cessation of antibiotics was associated with a significant decrease in antibiotic durations. This finding was confirmed in another meta-analysis, which showed that PCT-guided cessation was associated with a mean antibiotic duration of 7.35 days versus 8.85 days in the control arm −1.49 days (95% CI ·2.27–0.71, P<.001).[26]

Overall, serial evaluation of PCT in patients with sepsis is associated with significantly reduced 30-day mortality and may allow for a 1 to 3 day shorter duration of antimicrobial therapy with no apparent compromise in clinical outcomes. Of note, there are limitations with PCT as false positives and false negatives may be seen in some patient populations (**Table 9**).[24]

Methicillin-Resistant Staphylococcus aureus Nasal Screening

From 2011 to 2014, Staphylococcus aureus was the most prevalent pathogen implicated in VAP.[27] Although there are various methods to detect MRSA colonization, PCR assay has a faster turn-around time (<1 day) than site culture (1–3 days) and a higher sensitivity (92.5%) than culture (86.9%).[28] MRSA PCR testing detects mecA genetic sequencing, the gene responsible for methicillin resistance. Therefore, it is more likely to remain positive in patients already receiving antibiotic therapy than culture regardless of bacterial viability.[28]

Anti-MRSA therapy is often prescribed empirically for pneumonia in critically ill patients and de-escalated if MRSA is not isolated in a sputum or blood culture. However, there may be challenges with obtaining adequate respiratory cultures that may result in longer durations of broad-spectrum antimicrobial use, especially in non-intubated patients. Respiratory samples obtained after receipt of empiric antimicrobial therapy may have a lower yield in identifying a causative pathogen and also result in prolonged empiric regimens. Therefore, non-culture-based testing is an important tool for AMS de-escalation strategies.

Several studies have demonstrated high negative predictive values (NPV) of MRSA nares screening for MRSA pneumonia. One study out of the Veterans Affairs system evaluated MRSA nares colonization screening at admission and transfer and data from 561,325 cultures to determine NPV of MRSA screening in determination of subsequent positive MRSA culture. Overall, the NPV of MRSA nares screening for ruling out MRSA infection at any site of infection was 96.5% and 96.1% for respiratory infections.[29] A systematic review and meta-analysis confirmed a high NPV (96.5%) in pneumonia.[30]

Overall, MRSA nares screening has a high specificity and NPV for ruling out MRSA pneumonia. Although many studies used protocols to screen for MRSA in the nares at

ICU admission, with some repeating the screening weekly, Mallidi *and colleagues* demonstrated the NPV remained high (98%) even when using nares screens from within 60 days of hospital admission, indicating MRSA nares screening from a recent hospital admission may successfully guide empiric antimicrobial therapy in the ED and ICU settings.[31] When nares screening is negative for MRSA, it is reasonable to withhold or rapidly de-escalate anti-MRSA antimicrobial therapy.

CLINICS CARE POINTS

- Classification of pneumonia as either community-acquired or hospital-acquired will guide selection of empirical antimicrobial therapy.
- 5 to 7 days of treatment is generally sufficient to treat community-acquired pneumonia; however, procalcitonin may be a useful biomarker to support cessation of therapy sooner.
- Patients with hospital-acquired and ventilator-associated pneumonia should be risk-stratified for multidrug-resistant pathogens, with the cornerstone of therapy being a combination of anti-pseudomonal and anti-methicillin-resistant *Staphylococcus aureus* therapy.
- Immunocompromised patients should be managed on a case-by-case basis to ensure appropriate broad-spectrum antibiotics have been initiated to target certain pathogens.
- Collaboration with antimicrobial stewardship programs ensures optimization in overall antibiotic use while minimizing the risk of adverse effects from excessive antibiotic treatment (eg, *Clostridioides difficile* infection, development of antimicrobial resistance, and so forth)

REFERENCES

1. Olson G, Davis AM. Diagnosis and Treatment of Adults with Community-Acquired Pneumonia. JAMA 2020;323(9):885–6.
2. Nair GB, Niederman MS. Updates on community acquired pneumonia management in the ICU. Pharmacol Ther 2021;217:107663.
3. Ticona JH, Zaccone VM, McFarlane IM. Community-Acquired Pneumonia: A Focused Review. Am J Med Case Rep 2021;9(1):45–52.
4. Mandell LA, Wunderink RG, Anzueto A, et al. Infectious Diseases Society of America/American Thoracic Society consensus guidelines on the management of community-acquired pneumonia in adults. Clin Infect Dis 2007;44(suppl 2): S27–72.
5. Metlay JP, Waterer GW, Long AC, et al. Diagnosis and Treatment of Adults with Community-acquired Pneumonia. An Official Clinical Practice Guideline of the American Thoracic Society and Infectious Diseases Society of America. Am J Respir Crit Care Med 2019;200(7):e45–67.
6. Telles JP, Cieslinski J, Gasparetto J, et al. Efficacy of Ceftriaxone 1 g daily Versus 2 g daily for The Treatment of Community Acquired Pneumonia: A Systematic Review with Meta-Analysis. Expert Rev Anti-infective Ther 2019;17(7):501–10.
7. Hasegawa S, Sada R, Yaegashi M, et al. Adult Pneumonia Study Group-Japan. 1g versus 2 g daily intravenous ceftriaxone in the treatment of community onset pneumonia - a propensity score analysis of data from a Japanese multicenter registry. BMC Infect Dis 2019;19(1):1079.

8. Dimopoulos G, Matthaiou DK, Karageorgopoulos DE, et al. Short- versus long-course antibacterial therapy for community-acquired pneumonia: a meta-analysis. Drugs 2008;68:1841–54.
9. Li JZ, Winston LG, Moore DH, et al. Efficacy of short-course antibiotic regimens for community-acquired pneumonia: a meta-analysis. Am J Med 2007;120: 783–90.
10. Tansarli GS, Mylonakis E. Systematic review and meta-analysis of the efficacy of short-course antibiotic treatments for community-acquired pneumonia in adults. Antimicrob Agents Chemother 2018;62. e00635-18.
11. Kalil AC, Metersky ML, Klompas M, et al. Management of Adults With Hospital-acquired and Ventilator-associated Pneumonia: 2016 Clinical Practice Guidelines by the Infectious Diseases Society of America and the American Thoracic Society. Clin Infect Dis 2016;63(5):e61–111.
12. Torres A, Niederman MS, Chastre J, et al. International ERS/ESICM/ESCMID/ALAT guidelines for the management of hospital-acquired pneumonia and ventilator-associated pneumonia: Guidelines for the management of hospital-acquired pneumonia (HAP)/ventilator-associated pneumonia (VAP) of the European Respiratory Society (ERS), European Society of Intensive Care Medicine (ESICM), European Society of Clinical Microbiology and Infectious Diseases (ESCMID) and Asociación Latinoamericana del Tórax (ALAT). Eur Respir J 2017;50(3):1700582.
13. Berton DC, Kalil AC, Teixeira PJ. Quantitative versus qualitative cultures of respiratory secretions for clinical outcomes in patients with ventilator-associated pneumonia. Cochrane Database Syst Rev 2014;10:CD006482.
14. Wunderink RG, Srinivasan A, Barie PS, et al. Antibiotic Stewardship in the Intensive Care Unit. An Official American Thoracic Society Workshop Report in Collaboration with the AACN, CHEST, CDC, and SCCM. Ann Am Thorac Soc 2020; 17(5):531–40.
15. Luther MK, Timbrook TT, Caffrey AR, et al. Vancomycin Plus Piperacillin-Tazobactam and Acute Kidney Injury in Adults: A Systematic Review and Meta-Analysis. Crit Care Med 2018;46(1):12–20.
16. Guilhaumou R, Benaboud S, Bennis Y, et al. Optimization of the treatment with beta-lactam antibiotics in critically ill patients - Guidelines from the French Society of Pharmacology and Therapeutics (Société Française de Pharmacologie et Thérapeutique - SFPT) and the French Society of Anaesthesia. Crit Care 2019; 23(1):1–20.
17. Rybak MJ, Le J, Lodise TP, et al. Executive Summary: Therapeutic Monitoring of Vancomycin for Serious Methicillin-Resistant Staphylococcus aureus Infections: A Revised Consensus Guideline and Review of the American Society of Health-System Pharmacists, the Infectious Diseases Society of America, the Pediatric Infectious Diseases Society, and the Society of Infectious Diseases Pharmacists. Pharmacotherapy 2020;40(4):363–7.
18. Chastre J, Wolff M, Fagon JY, et al, PneumA Trial Group. Comparison of 8 vs 15 days of antibiotic therapy for ventilator-associated pneumonia in adults: a randomized trial. JAMA 2003;290(19):2588–98.
19. Pugh R, Grant C, Cooke RP, et al. Short-course versus prolonged-course antibiotic therapy for hospital-acquired pneumonia in critically ill adults. Cochrane Database Syst Rev 2015;2015(8):CD007577.
20. Dimopoulos G, Poulakou G, Pneumatikos IA, et al. Short- vs long-duration antibiotic regimens for ventilator-associated pneumonia: a systematic review and meta-analysis. Chest 2013;144(6):1759–67.

21. Ramirez JA, Musher DM, Evans SE, et al. Treatment of Community-Acquired Pneumonia in Immunocompromised Adults: A Consensus Statement Regarding Initial Strategies. Chest 2020;158(5):1896–911.

22. Blumenthal KG, Peter JG, Trubiano JA, et al. Antibiotic allergy. Lancet 2019; 393(10167):183–98.

23. Zagursky RJ, Pichichero ME. Cross-reactivity in β-Lactam Allergy. J Allergy Clin Immunol Pract 2018;6(1):72–81.e1.

24. Rhee C. Using Procalcitonin to Guide Antibiotic Therapy. Open Forum Infect Dis 2016;7(4):ofw249.

25. Lam SW, Bauer SR, Fowler R, et al. Systematic review and meta-analysis of procalcitonin-guidance versus usual care for antimicrobial management in critically ill patients: focus on subgroups based on antibiotic initiation, cessation, or mixed strategies. Crit Care Med 2018;46:684–90.

26. Iankova I, Thompson-Leduc P, Kirson NY, et al. Efficacy and safety of procalcitonin guidance in patients with suspected or confirmed sepsis: a systematic review and meta-analysis. Crit Care Med 2018;46:691–8.

27. Weiner LM, Webb AK, Limbago B, et al. Antimicrobial-resistant pathogens associated with healthcare-associated infections: summary of data reported to the National Healthcare Safety Network at the Centers for Disease Control and Prevention, 2011-2014. Infect Control Hosp Epidemiol 2016;37(11):1288–301.

28. Carr AL, Daley MJ, Givens Merkel K, et al. Clinical Utility of Methicillin-Resistant Staphylococcus aureus Nasal Screening for Antimicrobial Stewardship: A Review of Current Literature. Pharmacotherapy 2018;38:1216–28.

29. Mergenhagen KA, Starr KE, Wattengel BA, et al. Determining the Utility of Methicillin-Resistant Staphylococcus aureus Nares Screening in Antimicrobial Stewardship. Clin Infect Dis 2020;71:1142–8.

30. Parente DM, Cunha CB, Mylonakis E, et al. The Clinical Utility of Methicillin-Resistant Staphylococcus aureus (MRSA) Nasal Screening to Rule Out MRSA Pneumonia: A Diagnostic Meta-analysis With Antimicrobial Stewardship Implications. Clin Infect Dis 2018;67:1–7.

31. Mallidi MG, Slocum GW, Peksa GD, et al. Impact of Prior-to-Admission Methicillin-Resistant *Staphylococcus aureus* Nares Screening in Critically Ill Adults With Pneumonia. Ann Pharmacother 2022;56(2):124–30.

Right Ventricular Failure and Pulmonary Hypertension

Sara E. Crager, MD[a,b,*], Caroline Humphreys, MD[a]

KEYWORDS

- Right ventricular failure • Pulmonary hypertension • Cardiogenic shock
- Massive pulmonary embolism

KEY POINTS

- Right ventricular dysfunction plays a central role in high-risk, but relatively rare, conditions such as massive pulmonary embolism and primary pulmonary arterial hypertension; however, it also can be an important component of several disorders routinely encountered in the emergency department (ED) setting, including sepsis, adult respiratory distress syndrome, and chronic heart failure.
- Comorbid conditions frequently present in the ED population—such as COPD, methamphetamine abuse, and morbid obesity—are frequently associated with undiagnosed underlying pulmonary hypertension, and these patients may be particularly susceptible to the development of acute decompensated right ventricular failure when presenting with acute disorders that are independently associated with right ventricular dysfunction.
- Because the pathophysiology of acute decompensated right ventricular failure involves a cascade of superimposed vicious cycles that, once established, can be difficult to extricate from, avoiding diagnostic and management pitfalls in the ED becomes particularly important.
- Frequent diagnostic pitfalls include attributing lactic acidosis to septic rather than cardiogenic shock, ruling out cardiogenic shock based on observation of a hyperdynamic left ventricular function on bedside echo, and inferring the absence of volume overload based on normal-appearing lung fields on chest radiograph.
- Frequent management pitfalls include aggressive intravenous fluid administration, failure to support blood pressure by prompt initiation of appropriate vasopressors, and unnecessary endotracheal intubation.

The authors have nothing to disclose.
[a] Emergency Medicine, University of California Los Angeles, 924 Westwood Boulevard, Suite 300, Los Angeles, CA 90095, USA; [b] Critical Care Anesthesia, Los Angeles, CA, USA
* Corresponding author. Emergency Medicine, University of California Los Angeles, Los Angeles, CA.
E-mail address: sara.crager@gmail.com

INTRODUCTION

It is most useful for emergency providers (EPs) to approach pulmonary hypertension (PH) in the context of a broader understanding of right ventricular failure. Patients with known, chronic PH will constitute a minority of patients with right ventricular dysfunction (RVD) encountered in the emergency department (ED), and EPs will be best served by viewing PH as part of a spectrum of patients presenting with acute decompensated right ventricular failure (ADRVF).

EPs often regard PH and RVD as relatively rare entities that are mainly the province of specialists. In actuality, they are important components of the pathophysiology of several conditions frequently encountered in the ED:

- *Sepsis*: RVD is present in more than one-third of septic patients.[1] Although the presence of left ventricular (LV) systolic dysfunction does not seem to confer an increased risk of mortality, RVD seems to be associated with a 2- to 3-fold increase in mortality in patients with septic shock.[2]
- *Congestive heart failure (CHF)*: RVD is present in greater than 40% of patients with chronic left-sided heart failure and is a predictor of mortality in these patients.[3]
- *Chronic obstructive pulmonary disease (COPD)*: some degree of PH is present in approximately 20% of patients with COPD, and PH may occur in up to 90% of patients with severe COPD.[4]
- *Adult respiratory distress syndrome (ARDS)*: RVD is present in greater than 20% of patients with ARDS and is associated with a significantly increased risk of mortality.[5]
- *COVID*: in a recent meta-analysis, RVD was found to be present in 1 out of 5 patients hospitalized with COVID-19 and was associated with more than a 3-fold increase in mortality.[6]
- *Obesity hypoventilation syndrome*: greater than 50% of patients with obesity hypoventilation syndrome have PH,[7] and PH frequently goes undiagnosed in this population.[8]
- *Methamphetamine abuse*: a recent study of the national Pulmonary Hypertension Association Registry found that methamphetamine-associated PH accounted for greater than 20% of PH cases.[9]
- *Massive pulmonary embolus (PE)*: mortality in patients with massive PE is due to hemodynamic collapse from ADRVF, with most of the deaths occurring in the first 1 to 2 hours after presentation.[10]

Failure to recognize PH and/or RVD can become particularly problematic because routine interventions often performed early in a patient's ED course—such as intravenous fluid (IVF) administration and emergent endotracheal intubation (ETI)—have the potential to precipitate clinical deterioration in these patients. As such, it is important for EPs to become comfortable with early recognition and ED management of ADRVF; this is an area that lacks a robust body of evidence to guide management and instead relies on a solid understanding of the relevant pathophysiology.

PATHOPHYSIOLOGY
Right Ventricular Afterload

The systemic vascular resistance (SVR) constitutes the LV afterload, and the pulmonary vascular resistance (PVR) constitutes the RV afterload (**Fig. 1**). Pressures in the systemic and pulmonary circulations can fluctuate independently; the PVR can be elevated in the absence of SVR elevation and vice vera.

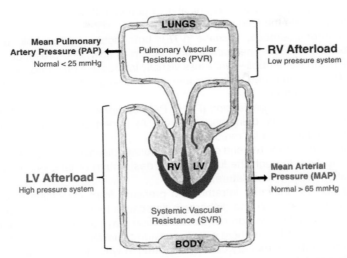

Fig. 1. Comparison of right and left ventricular afterload. The left side of the circulatory system is a high-pressure system, whereas the right side of the circulatory system is normally a low-pressure system. MAP, mean arterial pressure; PAP, pulmonary artery pressure; PVR, pulmonary vascular resistance; SVR, systemic vascular resistance.

Perhaps the most important thing to understand about the physiology of the RV is how it responds to afterload (**Fig. 2**).

- The muscular LV tolerates afterload well, with a minimal drop in stroke volume even in response to relatively large increases in SVR.
- The RV, on the other hand, is highly sensitive to increasing afterload, whereby even a small increase in PVR results in a precipitous decline in RV stroke volume.

The major factors driving elevations in RV afterload fall into 2 categories: obstructive and vasoconstrictive.

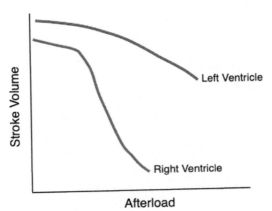

Fig. 2. Comparison of the left and right ventricular stroke volume in response to increasing afterload.

Obstructive: major causes of mechanical obstruction to flow through the pulmonary circulation include the following:

1. *Venous thromboembolic disease (VTE)*: both acute and chronic pulmonary thromboemboli cause mechanical obstruction to flow. The presence of a large volume of smaller emboli—while less visually impressive on computed tomography (CT) scan compared with a saddle embolus—can still cause significant mechanical obstruction.
2. *Pulmonary arterial hypertension (PAH)*: PAH comprises a subset of PH causes arising from primary pulmonary artery (PA) hypertrophy due to endothelial dysfunction and vascular remodeling.
3. *Lung disease*: both acute and chronic pulmonary disease can cause obstruction of forward flow through the lungs due to destruction of lung parenchyma and obliteration of lung vasculature.
4. *Morbid obesity*: elevated intrathoracic pressure from excessive weight compressing the chest wall and diaphragm can cause functional restrictive lung.

Vasoconstrictive: although adrenergic stimulation plays a role in regulation of pulmonary vasoconstriction, there are several additional factors that affect the vasomotor tone of the pulmonary circulation, often in ways that are distinct from the systemic circulation:

1. *Hypoxemia*: hypoxemia triggers pulmonary vasoconstriction in order to optimize ventilation perfusion matching (**Fig. 3**). A "side effect" of this vasoconstrictor response is elevated PVR associated with hypoxemia.
2. *Hypercarbia and acidemia*: pulmonary vasoconstriction is enhanced by both hypercapnia and acidemia (**Fig. 4**).
3. *Inflammation*: in contrast to the systemic circulation—in which the predominant vasomotor response to inflammation is vasodilation—release of inflammatory mediators into the pulmonary circulation triggers pulmonary vasoconstriction. Pulmonary vasoconstriction in response to cytokines released by activated platelets plays a significant role in the pathogenesis of massive PE.

Obstructive and vasoconstrictive mechanisms act synergistically, whereby obstructive causes tend to promote the development of vasoconstrictive causes, which can

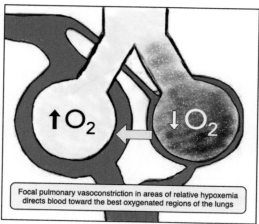

Focal pulmonary vasoconstriction in areas of relative hypoxemia directs blood toward the best oxygenated regions of the lungs

Fig. 3. Hypoxic pulmonary vasoconstriction. As a consequence of this phenomenon, hypoxia causes increases in pulmonary vascular resistance.

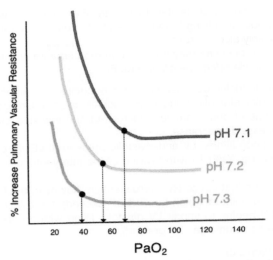

Fig. 4. Pulmonary vasoconstriction in response to hypoxemia and acidemia. Hypoxemia causes a "dose-dependent" increase in pulmonary vascular resistance, which is magnified in the presence of acidemia.

then promote the development of vascular remodeling and thrombosis that subsequently exacerbate obstructive causes.

Right Ventricular Preload

The RV is a significantly more compliant structure than the LV, with large changes in volume resulting in relatively small changes in pressure. Consequently, at the lower end of the volume spectrum, the RV is preload dependent insofar, as it relies on adequate intravascular volume to maintain right-sided filling pressures sufficient to sustain cardiac output (CO). Once, however, volume loading reaches the point at which further increases in RV volume result in significant increases in RV pressure; the RV–by the same token of its relatively high compliance–can rapidly become overdistended.

The point at which this occurs highly depends on whether the RV afterload is normal or elevated. Regardless, once RV overdistension begins to occur, several sequelae arising from RV dilation ensue that, together, can precipitate ADRVF in patients with or without underlying PH or RVD:

1. Impaired ability of the RV to generate contractile force due to the mechanical effect on myocytes of overstretching the RV free wall.
2. Elevated RV wall tension that simultaneously results in a reduction in coronary filling and increased oxygen demand, making the RV more susceptible to ischemic insult.
3. Tricuspid annular dilation that can precipitate or exacerbate existing tricuspid regurgitation, contributing to worsening RV volume overload and overdistension.
4. Reduction of LV preload that arises from interventricular septal shift, as discussed later.

Ventricular Interdependence

The functional interplay between the LV and the RV involves both in-series and in-parallel interactions.

Series interaction: in order of maintain LV CO, the RV CO must match that of the LV. When RV forward flow supplying blood to the LV decreases, LV forward flow to the body must necessarily also decrease.

Parallel interaction: because they share a common septum, volume and pressure changes in one ventricle affect the other (**Fig. 5**).

- Because the ventricles co-exist within the nondistensible space of the pericardium, ventricular diastolic filling is functionally a zero-sum-game: if the end-diastolic volume of one ventricle is increased, the end-diastolic volume of the other will necessarily decrease.
- Under normal conditions, LV end-diastolic pressure (LVEDP) exceeds RV end-diastolic pressure (RVEDP) with bowing of the interventricular septum into the RV.
- Under conditions that cause RV overdistention, however, the RVEDP begins to increase. At the point at which the RVEDP exceeds the LVEDP, septal bowing toward the LV begins to impair LV diastolic filling with a concomitant drop in LV end-diastolic volume (ie,: LV preload).

Right Ventricular Perfusion

Recall that tissue perfusion is not determined by blood pressure alone, but rather by a pressure *gradient* (**Fig. 6**).

- LV systolic pressures, by definition, approach systemic systolic blood pressure. Because of the absence of a pressure gradient between the LV and coronary arteries during systole, most of the LV perfusion occurs during diastole.

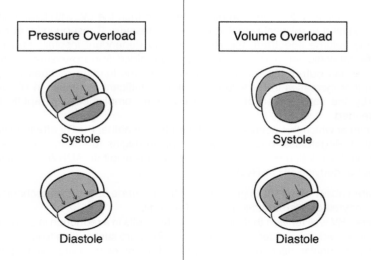

Fig. 5. Comparison of interventricular septal shift under conditions of pressure overload versus isolated volume overload. Echocardiographic appearance on parasternal short view of the RV (*blue*) and the LV (*red*) during systole and diastole under conditions of either right ventricular pressure overload versus right ventricular volume overload. Depending on the severity of volume overload and the degree and chronicity of pressure overload, right ventricular dilation may or may not be observed. A chronic pressure-overloaded RV. LV, left ventricle; RV, right ventricle.

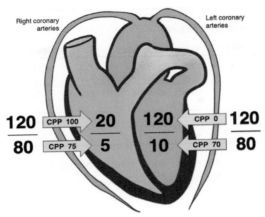

Fig. 6. Comparison of perfusion of the right and left ventricles throughout the cardiac cycle. CPP, coronary perfusion pressure.

- The right heart, in contrast, is a low-pressure system. Consequently, there is a robust gradient between the coronary artery pressure and RV pressure during both diastole *and* systole, providing continuous perfusion to the RV throughout the cardiac cycle with most of the perfusion occurring during systole when the pressure gradient is greatest.

Causes of Right Ventricular Failure

Causes of RV failure in acutely ill patients may be divided into 3 categories (**Table 1**): pressure overload, volume overload, and decreased contractility.

Pressure overload: RV pressure overload can occur acutely or chronically. When exposed to chronic elevations in afterload, RV remodeling occurs such that the RV begins to resemble the more muscular LV and is thereby able to better sustain forward flow even in the context of even significantly increased afterload.

Causes of RV pressure overload are generally broken down into categories using the World Health Organization PH Groups system and detailed in **Table 2**.

Volume overload: RV volume overload can occur in patients both with and without chronic PH and/or RVD.

Patients with chronic disease: patients with chronic PH may be compensated from a pressure loading standpoint; however, they generally require diuretic management to maintain a steady state. In failures to maintain euvolemia–often in the context of worsening renal function and/or medication noncompliance–these patients can present with ADRVF due to volume overload.

Patients without chronic disease: ADRVF due to volume overload in the absence of chronic disease is most often iatrogenic.

- This may occur in the settings such as massive PE, when the clinician either fail to recognize the underlying cause of acute deterioration and/or has misconceptions regarding the utility of fluid administration in patients with ADRVF due to increased afterload.
- Even in the absence of elevated RV afterload, excessive volume loading can precipitate RVD once volume administration reaches the point of cause RV overdistention and progressive dilation, as discussed earlier.

Table 1		
Major causes of right ventricular failure		
Pressure Overload	**Volume Overload**	**Depressed Contractility**
Thromboembolic disease	Excessive fluid administration	Right ventricular myocardial ischemia
Primary pulmonary arterial hypertension	Insufficient diuresis	Myocarditis
Lung disease	—	Sepsis
Morbid obesity	—	—

Depressed contractility: the major acute causes of isolated RV contractile depression are essentially similar to those of the LV:

1. Myocardial ischemia
2. Myocarditis
3. Septic cardiomyopathy

It is notable that the septal component of LV contraction is a significant contributor to the ability of the RV to generate systolic pressures; as such, RV contractile dysfunction that occurs in concert with LV dysfunction can be particularly profound.

Pathophysiology of Acute Decompensated Right Ventricular Failure

The pathophysiology of acute decompensated RV failure is outlined in **Fig. 7** and may best be conceptualized as a cascade of superimposed vicious cycles, that, once established, can be difficult to extricate from. Any of the 3 etiologic categories mentioned earlier can act as entry points to the vicious cycle of acute decompensated RV failure. It is also important to note that multiple sequala of ETI—including systemic hypotension, hypoxemia, hypercarbia, and positive pressure ventilation—can act as vicious cycle precipitants, and the potential for simultaneous occurrence of 2 or more of these factors places patients with PH and/or RVD at high risk for dramatic hemodynamic deterioration during ETI. In one study of patients taken to the operating room for pulmonary embolectomy, hemodynamic collapse occurred in nearly 20% of patients during ETI.[11]

CLINICAL PRESENTATION AND EVALUATION
Types of Presentations

Major precipitants of acute RV failure in patients without any prior history of RVD or PH include the following:

- *Massive PE*: although it is a common misconception that "massive" refers to the thrombus size, massive PE is in fact defined by hemodynamic instability due to ADRVF as a consequence of acute VTE.
- *COVID-19*: acute presentations of patients with COVID with abrupt hemodynamic deterioration triggered by ADRVF in the *absence* of massive PE are increasingly being reported.[12]
- *RV myocardial infarction (RVMI)*: isolated RVMI is relatively rare and most often associated with acute MI of the LV inferior wall.
- *Myocarditis*: although biventricular involvement is common, isolated RV myocarditis is exceptionally rare.
- *Left ventricular assist device (LVAD)*: there is a high rate of RV failure in LVAD patients with multifactorial mechanisms consequent to derangements in both the series and parallel interactions between the RV and LV.

Table 2
Classification of pulmonary hypertension

	Group	Pathogenesis	Common Causes
1	Primary pulmonary arterial hypertension	• Increased pulmonary vascular resistance due to intrinsic disease of the pulmonary arterial vasculature • Associated with endothelial dysfunction and hyperplasia similar to that seen with systemic essential hypertension	Connective tissue & autoimmune disease (scleroderma, SLE, RA) Drugs and toxins (methamphetamine, fenfluramine, dasatinib) Portal hypertension Infectious (HIV, schistosomiasis) Idiopathic and heritable
2	PH due to left heart disease	• Chronic elevations in venous back pressure from left heart failure • May develop secondary vascular remodeling that can resemble intrinsic disease	LV systolic dysfunction LV diastolic dysfunction Mitral regurgitation & stenosis Aortic regurgitation & stenosis
3	PH due to chronic lung disease	• Chronic hypoxic pulmonary vasoconstriction • Ultimately results in vascular remodeling	COPD ILD OSA Obesity hypoventilation syndrome
4	PH due to chronic thromboembolic disease	• Mechanical obstruction of the pulmonary arterial vasculature	Chronic thromboembolic disease Intrathoracic tumors
5	Multifactorial PH	• Potpourri of mechanisms	Myeloproliferative disease Sickle cell disease Sarcoidosis Hyperthyroidism (primarily toxic multinodular goiter)

Abbreviations: COPD, chronic obstructive pulmonary disease; HIV, human immunodeficiency virus; ILD, interstitial lung disease; LV, left ventricle; OSA, obstructive sleep apnea; PH, pulmonary hypertension; PVR, pulmonary vascular resistance; RA, rheumatoid arthritis; SLE, systemic lupus erythematosus.

Although patients may present acutely with truly de novo ADRVF, it is more common to see acute or chronic presentations whereby some degree of underlying pulmonary vascular disease is exacerbated by 1 of the 3 main causes of RV failure detailed earlier.

Many patients may have undiagnosed underlying PH and/or RVD, making it more difficult to rapidly identify ADRVF as their primary problem in the acute setting. Specific scenarios that should raise suspicion include the following:

- Morbid obesity, especially when associated with obesity hypoventilation syndrome and/or obstructive sleep apnea
- Severe COPD or interstitial lung disease
- Methamphetamine use

In patients with an established diagnosis of PH and/or RVD, the major clinical question becomes the identification of factors that may have provoked an acute decompensation. Frequent precipitants include the following:

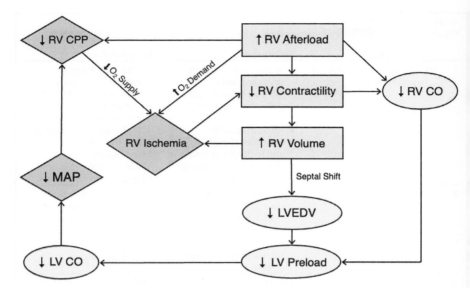

Fig. 7. Vicious cycle pathophysiology of acute decompensated right ventricular failure. Because of the inability of the RV to maintain normal contractility in response to even relatively small increases in afterload (see **Fig. 3**), a frequent entry point into this vicious cycle is an increase in RV afterload. As RV stroke volume decreases, RV volume begins to increase, as blood backs up into the RV. This increasing RV volume eventually leads to progressively worsening interventricular septal shift, which ultimately compromises LV filling (see **Fig. 6**). The associated drop in LVEDV in combination with low RV CO due to depressed RV contractility and/or increased RV afterload can dramatically decrease LV preload, at which point LV CO will start to decrease. Systemic hypotension ensues, decreasing RV coronary perfusion. The RV CPP takes a second hit if elevated RV systolic pressures associated with high RV afterload are simultaneously present (see **Fig. 1**). Depressed RV CPP compromises RV oxygen supply and precipitates the development of worsening ischemia, even in the absence of primary coronary artery pathology; the resultant RV ischemia can be particularly profound if the drop in RV oxygen supply occurs concurrently with increased oxygen demand associated with elevated RV wall tension due to RV volume and/or pressure overload. Global RV ischemia further contributes to worsening RV contractility, perpetuating the vicious cycle. CO, cardiac output; CPP, coronary perfusion pressure; LV, left ventricle; LVEDV, left ventricular end-diastolic volume; MAP, mean arterial pressure; RV, right ventricle.

- Interruption of pulmonary vasodilator medications (eg: sildenafil, Remodulin).
- Volume overload due to noncompliance with diuretic therapy and/or worsening renal function.
- Exacerbation of underlying primary pulmonary disease.
- PH predisposes to the formation of *in situ* PEs due to slow flow through the PA, and patients with underlying RVD may not have the physiologic reserve to tolerate even relatively small thromboemboli.

History and Physical Examination

Signs and symptoms: patients with RV failure do not necessarily present with what are thought of as "classic" symptoms of heart failure.

- The lung examination is generally normal in the absence of concomitant LV failure or chronic lung disease.
- Patients often present with abdominal pain or distention in the context of congestive hepatopathy due to elevated right heart pressures being transmitted to the portal venous system and may even present with mesenteric ischemia secondary to a combination of increased back pressures due to mesenteric venous congestion combined with decreased forward flow from concomitant cardiogenic shock.
- Prominent jugular venous pressure elevations as well as peripheral edema may be present, although it is important to note that absence of these signs does not rule out ADRVF, particularly if acute in onset.

Patients will often present tachypneic, tachycardic and, not infrequently, hypoxemic. Particularly given the significant risks associated with ETI in these patients, it is crucial to understand that their oxygen saturation (SpO_2) may be low due to several possible mechanisms, most of which are likely to be exacerbated rather than alleviated by ETI:

- *Massive PE*: hypoxemia in massive PE is not due to dysfunction of the pulmonary parenchyma (eg: pulmonary edema, pneumonia, and so forth) but rather due to VQ mismatch and global tissue hypoperfusion, neither of which will be improved by ETI.
- *Chronic lung disease*: patients with PH due to chronic lung disease often have a baseline low SpO_2. It can be extremely challenging to assess whether their acute presentation is due primarily to an exacerbation of their chronic lung disease as opposed to the development of ADRVF in the context of chronic PH. Regardless, attempting aggressive treatment that simultaneously address both possibilities is prudent before considering ETI.
- *Falsely low SpO2 reading*: patients presenting in cardiogenic shock not infrequently have spuriously low SpO_2 readings due to decreased peripheral perfusion. In contrast to patients with LV failure, patients with cardiogenic shock due to ADRVF are unlikely to have pulmonary edema, and it is therefore important to identify spurious SpO_2 values early, as that ongoing concern for hypoxemia could trigger an unnecessary ETI, which can precipitate acute hemodynamic collapse in these patients.

Past medical history (PMH): the key details of PMH specific to patients with PH and RVD include the following:

- *Disease history*: establish if the patient has a known PMH of RVD or PH and, if so, whether they are listed for transplant or undergoing a transplant evaluation. The latter may help inform decisions about whether transfer for possible extracorporeal membrane oxygenation may be reasonable in cases of refractory ADRVF.
- *Medication history*: this should focus on 3 different categories:
  1. Pulmonary vasodilators that are associated with rebound PH when acutely discontinued (eg,: sildenafil, Remodulin).
  2. Oral anticoagulant use in the absence of other obvious indications suggests severe enough PH to warrant prophylaxis for in situ PE.
  3. Loop diuretic use and home doses to help guide initial dosing of furosemide and/or bumetanide if diuresis becomes necessary.
- *Diagnostic studies*: some patients will have a prior right heart catheterization with direct measurement of PA pressures; more commonly patients may have a previous echocardiogram documenting a PA systolic pressure. Information on

baseline PA pressures is useful both to help determine disease severity as well as to help guide mean arterial pressure (MAP) goals (see later discussion on systemic blood pressure targets).

Laboratory Findings and Imaging

Laboratory findings: the main challenge in the laboratory workup of patients presenting with ADRVF is to avoid misinterpretation of commonly acquired laboratory findings. Laboratory findings in ADRVF are often misconstrued as consistent with septic or hypovolemic shock rather than cardiogenic shock due to ADRVF, which increase the likelihood of clinically significant errors in management.

- *Lactate*: it is a common misconception that lactic acidosis is synonymous with septic shock. Lactic acidosis in fact can be associated with any shock state, including cardiogenic shock due to ADRVF. Recall that fluid administration will only improve a lactic acidosis if volume administration improves tissue perfusion, which is not the case when the cause of tissue hypoperfusion is cardiogenic shock.
- *Renal function tests*: patients will often present with acute kidney injury (AKI) due to renal hypoperfusion secondary to ADRVF. An elevated BUN/Cr ratio that suggests a prerenal cause can be particularly confusing in this context because prerenal AKI is often misinterpreted as synonymous with hypovolemia. In reality, however, a prerenal AKI simply indicates that the kidneys are receiving insufficient forward flow but does not signify whether the underlying cause of this insufficient forward flow is hypovolemic, distributive, or cardiogenic.
- *Liver function tests (LFTs)*: it is not necessary to obtain LFTs, but, if obtained, patients may have a transaminitis due to congestive hepatopathy, which can be misinterpreted as evidence of an RUQ process causing abdominal sepsis, particularly in patients presenting with abdominal pain.
- *Brain natriuretic peptide (BNP)*: BNP can be spuriously low in patients with morbid obesity; this may be problematic in patients with PH secondary to obesity hypoventilation syndrome insofar, as a false-negative BNP may lead to incorrect conclusions regarding the presence of heart failure and/or volume overload.
- *Troponin*: in the absence of electrocardiogram finding that suggests acute inferior and/or posterior ischemia, a positive troponin likely indicates demand ischemia rather than coronary artery occlusion.
- *Arterial blood gas (ABG)*: an ABG can be particularly useful in these patients, especially if there is any question regarding the accuracy of SpO_2 readings. In addition, CO_2 and pH are useful with regard to identification of potentially modifiable factors that may be contributing to increased pulmonary vasoconstriction.

Imaging: chest radiograph may show an enlarged cardiac silhouette but is often normal in the absence of concomitant LV failure or primary lung disease. In addition to ruling out PE, CT angiography (CTA) of the chest can provide a better assessment of RV size as well as underlying lung disease. Reflux of IV contrast into the interior vena cava and/or hepatic vein on CTA is a specific—although insensitive—sign that suggests ADRVF.

Point-of-care ultrasound (POCUS): a frequent pitfall in patients with ADRVF is that the LV often seems hyperdynamic; this is not due to systemic hypovolemia, but rather due to poor RV CO. As such, an underfilled-appearing LV should always trigger evaluation for the presence of RV dilation and septal flattening that suggests ADRVF (see **Fig. 6**). Visual estimation of RV systolic function is not straightforward and should not be used to draw firm clinical conclusions on POCUS. Observation of an abnormally thick-walled RV may suggest a PH with a chronically pressure-overloaded RV.

EMERGENCY CRITICAL CARE MANAGEMENT

RVD and PH are areas that lack a robust body of evidence to guide management, and instead rely on a thorough understanding of related pathophysiology and knowledge of expert opinion, coupled with meticulous clinical attentiveness at the bedside.

There are 5 key management components (**Table 3**):

1. Optimize volume status
2. Support systemic blood pressure
3. Decrease right ventricular afterload
4. Support right ventricular contractility
5. Caution with ETI

Optimize Volume Status

The RV response to volume loading highly depends on whether RV afterload is normal or elevated.

Normal RV afterload: in the setting of normal RV afterload, ADRVF due to contractile dysfunction may result in a "preload-dependent" RV requiring volume augmentation in order to maintain CO. The clinical relevance of this physiologic principle, however, is unclear:

- Based on this presumptive physiology and a single study of 28 patients conducted in 1989, the American Heart Association guidelines continue to state that nitrates are contraindicated in RVMI.[13] In contrast, more recent studies—collectively comprising greater than 1000 patients—found no increased risk of adverse events associated with nitrate administration in patients with acute RVMI.[13]
- The reported efficacy of volume administration in RVMI is variable.[14] Expert opinion suggests careful volume administration in patients with an RVMI presenting with hypotension via aliquots of 200 to 300 mL of crystalloid with serial reassessment of clinical effect.[15]

Elevated RV afterload: when RV failure occurs in the setting of increased RV afterload, intravascular volume expansion can precipitate rapid clinical deterioration and should be avoided. Volume removal is often a critical part of management in these patients.

- Patients with underlying chronic RVD or PH are often volume overloaded on initial presentation. Even in the case of acute PE—in which there is no expectation that these patients would be necessarily hypervolemic at presentation—a single furosemide bolus on admission seems to produce significant and earlier improvements in RV function compared with IVF administration, without any associated adverse events.[16] Certainly in patients presenting with massive PE who have been administered IVF during their initial ED course and are decompensating hemodynamically, it would be reasonable to initiate diuresis to at least restore euvolemia.

It is critical to understand that diuresis may be required even in the presence of AKI. AKI in the context of cardiogenic shock due to ADRVF is generally due to cardiorenal syndrome and can only be successfully addressed by improving forward flow to optimize renal perfusion, which generally requires volume removal.

- In patients with elevated RV afterload, the combination of septal shift due to elevated RV pressures and decreased volume delivery to the LV due to

Table 3
Critical management components of acute decompensated right ventricular failure

Critical Management Priorities	
Optimize fluid status	• Volume administration can precipitate clinical deterioration in patients with elevated RV afterload • Patients with chronic PH and/or RVD often require diuresis • In patient with depressed RV contractility and normal RV afterload, may consider gentle volume boluses with frequent reassessments
Support systemic blood pressure	• Even transient hypotension can be problematic; low threshold to initiate early vasopressors and invasive blood pressure monitoring • Vasopressin and epinephrine are optimal, norepinephrine is also reasonable • Patients with elevated PA pressures may require higher MAP targets to optimize RV coronary perfusion pressures
Decrease RV afterload	• Correct of hypoxemia, hypercarbia, and acidemia • Initiation of an inhaled pulmonary vasodilator
Support RV contractility	• After correction of systemic hypotension, consider additional inotropic support particularly if failing to respond to diuretic challenge • Epinephrine is a reasonable first-line inotrope, can also consider addition of milrinone vs dobutamine if systemic blood pressures have normalized
Extreme caution with intubation	• High risk of hemodynamic deterioration with ETI • ETI rarely has a role in the management of patients whose acute decompensation is due *primarily* to ADRVF; if ETI is required as appropriate management for an acute condition in a patient with *comorbid* PH and/or RVD, it should be undertaken with careful hemodynamic management

Abbreviations: ADRVF, acute decompensated right ventricular failure; ETI, endotracheal intubation; MAP, mean arterial pressure; PA, pulmonary artery; PH, pulmonary hypertension; RV, right ventricle; RVD, right ventricular dysfunction.

depressed RV CO may lead to near obliteration of the LV at end-systole. In this circumstance additional volume loading has actually been shown to *decrease* LV preload.[17,18] Furthermore, worsening RV dilation precipitated by IVF administration increases RV transmural pressure and oxygen demand, thereby worsening RV ischemia.

• It is also important to note that in the case of ADRVF due to either pressure or volume overload, hypotension is not necessarily a contraindication to volume removal; due to the physiology of ADRVF in the context of elevated pulmonary pressures, volume removal may be expected to actually improve blood pressure by increasing CO, whereas volume administration is in fact likely to worsen hypotension as per the mechanisms outlined earlier.

• It is, however, the case that an initial diuretic challenge may not be successful because the kidneys are unlikely to respond robustly to diuretics in the absence of sufficient renal perfusion. As such, hemodynamic interventions to support systemic blood pressures and optimize RV function are often necessary preconditions to facilitate volume removal. Furthermore, because the RV has a flatter

Starling curve than the LV, a considerable amount of volume unloading may be necessary before any improvement in RV function is seen.[19] Once sufficient hemodynamic optimization occurs with associated improvements in renal perfusion, a "virtuous cycle" of RV volume offloading often begins, at which point significant increases in urine output may occur in a relatively short amount of time.

Approach to volume removal: early placement of a Foley catheter is recommended to monitor hourly urine output in order to guide prompt escalation of diuretic therapy.

- Diuresis may be initiated with a loop-diuretic bolus, followed by rapid dose escalation if an adequate response is not observed. Intravenous administration is preferred, as that severe mesenteric venous congestion may compromise intestinal perfusion in these patients. If there continues to be a suboptimal response to escalating doses of loop-diuretics, then it is reasonable to add chlorothiazide, and initiation of a furosemide or bumetanide drip may also be considered.
- If the patient still fails to respond, then further optimization renal perfusion may be accomplished by adding an inhaled pulmonary vasodilator if not already initiated, and it is also reasonable to consider initiation of additional RV inotropic support at this point.

Support Systemic Blood Pressure

Blood pressure targets: the RV is particularly prone to ischemia when RV coronary perfusion is hit with the dual insult of elevated pulmonary pressures occurring concurrently with systemic hypotension.

- Even relatively transient hypotension can act as a trigger for the vicious cycle of ADRVF; there should be a low threshold for pressor initiation and placement of an arterial line.
- To preserve the pressure gradient between the coronary arteries and the pressure-overloaded RV, it may be necessary to maintain systemic pressures higher than an MAP goal of 65; this is particularly important in patients with chronic PH, in whom RV systolic pressures may approach systemic pressures. Prior documentation of PA pressures can be helpful to guide MAP goals in these patients.

Pressor selection: as discussed earlier, in patients with elevated RH pressures, volume administration is unlikely to improve hypotension, and pressors are the mainstay of treatment. The ideal vasopressor for use in acute RV failure would be an agent that increases systemic blood pressure without increasing pulmonary pressures. In this context, pressor choice may be based on the degree to which a given pressures is associated with favorable effects on the PVR to SVR ratio. See **Fig. 8** for a comparison of vasoactives in the management of ADRVF.[20,21]

Decrease Right Ventricular Afterload

Correct hypoxemia, hypercapnia, and acidemia: these factors act both independently and synergistically to increase pulmonary vasoconstriction such that even if correction of all 3 is not possible, correction of even one of these variables will have disproportionally beneficial effects on pulmonary vasoconstriction (see **Fig. 5**).

Pulmonary vasodilators: pulmonary vasodilators may be administered systemically or via inhalation.

- *Systemic pulmonary vasodilators*: the major side effect of oral or intravenous administration of pulmonary vasodilators is systemic hypotension. Abrupt discontinuation of these medications should be avoided in the ED, if at all possible. If a patient who is taking chronic systemic pulmonary vasodilators presents with hypotension, the MAP should be supported with vasopressors while awaiting more definitive intensive care unit management. Alternatively or in addition, an inhaled pulmonary vasodilator may be initiated as a temporizing measure.
- *Inhaled pulmonary vasodilators*: the advantage of inhaled pulmonary vasodilators is that they rapidly induce pulmonary vasodilation and decrease PVR with relatively minimal effects on systemic blood pressure. Inhaled pulmonary vasodilators may be administered through ETI, high-flow nasal cannula, or—in some cases—venturi mask. At centers where it is not possible to initiate epoprostenol or nitric oxide through specialized continuous inhalational devices, off-label use of inhaled milrinone[22] or nitroglycerin[23] may be considered (**Table 4**).

Inotropic Support

Once RV perfusion has been improved through the correction of systemic hypotension and measures to decrease RV afterload have been undertaken, inotropes to support RV contractility may be initiated (see **Fig. 8**). In cases of PH due to LV failure, inotropes carry the additional benefit of improving LV forward flow, thereby decreasing RV afterload as well as indirectly improving RV contractility through augmentation of the role of the septum. Epinephrine is a reasonable first-line inotrope in patients who continue to have borderline low MAPs and/or escalating vasopressor requirements. In patients whose MAPs have normalized and are on stable vasopressor doses, dobutamine or milrinone may also be considered, particularly in the context of an inadequate response to diuresis due to suboptimal renal perfusion.

Caution with Endotracheal Intubation

The most important consideration regarding ETI is not selection of periintubation medications, but rather the decision of whether a patient truly requires intubation in the first

Drug	PVR	SVR	PVR : SVR	Comments
Vasopressin	↔ ↓	↑↑	↓↓	• Probably ideal first-line vasopressor to support systemic blood pressure for acute decompensated RV failure • Not titratable, so may need to add additional vasoactive medications.
Epinephrine	↓	↑	↓	• Can be useful as a single agent to support both RV contractility and systemic blood pressure • β1 and β2 effects more prominent than α1 effects at doses less than ~20mcg/min • Increasingly prominent α1 effects at higher doses.
Norepinephrine	↔ ↑	↑↑	↔	• Without the β2 to balance out the α1 effects on the pulmonary circulation, higher risk for pulmonary vasoconstriction, particularly at high doses
Phenylephrine	↑↑	↑↑	↑↑	• Suboptimal due to effect on PVR:SVR ratio
Dopamine	↑↑	↑↑	↑↑	• Suboptimal due to effect on PVR:SVR ratio • Risk of tachydysrhythmias
Dobutamine	↓↓	↓	↓↓	• Supports RV contractility and can decrease PVR • Can cause systemic hypotension and so may not be ideal during initial resuscitation • Risk of tachydysrhythmias
Milrinone	↓↓	↓	↓↓	• Supports RV contractility and decreases PVR • Can cause systemic hypotension so may not be ideal during initial resuscitation, particularly given the significantly longer on-off time compared to other vasoactive • Useful addition in patients who continue to have inadequate perfusion once systemic blood pressure has stabilized

Fig. 8. Comparison of vasoactive medications in the management of acute decompensated right ventricular failure.

Table 4
Inhaled pulmonary vasodilators

Drug	Route of Administration	Dose
Epoprostenol (*Brand names: Flolan, Veletri*)	Continuous inhalation via ETT or HFNC	0.05 mcg/kg/min
Nitric oxide	Continuous inhalation via ETT or HFNC	20 ppm
Milrinone	Intermittent inhalation via venturi mask	Concentration: 1 mg/mL Inhale 5 mg over 15–30 min
Nitroglycerin	Intermittent inhalation via venturi mask	Concentration: 1 mg/mL Inhale 5 mg over 15–30 min

place. Although ETI may be required as part of appropriate management of various acute conditions in patients with *comorbid* RVD or PH, ETI rarely has a role in the management of patients who are acutely ill *because* of ADRVF. Making this distinction necessitates both recognition of cases when ADRVF is the primary factor driving a patient's acute presentation, as well as the understanding that ETI is unlikely to be of benefit in this situation and in fact has significant potential to cause precipitous clinical deterioration in patients with ADRVF. The details of periintubation management of patients with comorbid RVD and/or PH requiring ETI has been discussed elsewhere.[24]

SUMMARY

Although RVD plays a central role in high-risk, but relatively rare, conditions such as massive PE and chronic PAH, it is also an important—if frequently unrecognized—component of several disorders routinely encountered in the ED setting such as sepsis, ARDS, and CHF. Comorbid conditions frequently present in the ED population, such as morbid obesity, COPD, and methamphetamine abuse, are not infrequently associated with undiagnosed underlying PH, and these patients may be particularly susceptible to the development of ADRVF when presenting with acute disorders that are independently associated with RVD. ADRFV may be easily mistaken for entities such as abdominal sepsis or septic shock, and a high index of suspicion in the appropriate clinical setting is required to avoid common pitfalls in the recognition of evolving ADRVF.

It is important for emergency physicians to understand the pathophysiology of ADRVF in order to avoid common management pitfalls that can result in significant morbidity and mortality, including aggressive IV fluid administration, failure to support blood pressure by prompt initiation of appropriate vasopressors, and unnecessary ETI.

Early diagnosis and appropriate management of PH and RVD by EPs has the potential to profoundly affect a patient's clinical course and can mean the difference between a routine admission of a hemodynamically stable patient and that same patient going into cardiac arrest in the ED.

REFERENCES

1. Vallabhajosyula S, Shankar A, Vojjini R, et al. Impact of right ventricular dysfunction on short-term and long-term mortality in sepsis: a meta-analysis of 1,373 patients. CHEST 2021;159:2254–63.
2. Lanspa MJ, Cirulis M, Wiley BM, et al. Right ventricular dysfunction in early sepsis and septic shock. Chest 2021;159:1055–63.

3. Iglesias-Garriz I, Olalla-Gómez C, Garrote C, et al. Contribution of right ventricular dysfunction to heart failure mortality: a meta-analysis. Rev Cardiovasc Med 2012; 13:e62–9.

4. Opitz I, Ulrich S. Pulmonary hypertension in chronic obstructive pulmonary disease and emphysema patients: prevalence, therapeutic options and pulmonary circulatory effects of lung volume reduction surgery. J Thorac Dis 2018;10: S2763–74.

5. Sato R, Dugar S, Cheungpasitporn W, et al. The impact of right ventricular injury on the mortality in patients with acute respiratory distress syndrome: a systematic review and meta-analysis. Crit Care 2021;25:172.

6. Corica B, Marra AM, Basili S, et al. Prevalence of right ventricular dysfunction and impact on all-cause death in hospitalized patients with COVID-19: a systematic review and meta-analysis. Sci Rep 2021;11:17774.

7. Almeneessier AS, Nashwan SZ, Al-Shamiri MQ, et al. The prevalence of pulmonary hypertension in patients with obesity hypoventilation syndrome: a prospective observational study. J Thorac Dis 2017;9:779–88.

8. Piper AJ, Lau EM. Positive Airway Pressure in Obesity Hypoventilation: Getting to the Heart of the Matter. Am J Respir Crit Care Med 2020;201:509–11.

9. Kolaitis NA, Zamanian RT, de Jesus Perez VA, et al. Clinical differences and outcomes between methamphetamine-associated and idiopathic pulmonary arterial hypertension in the pulmonary hypertension association registry. Ann Am Thorac Soc 2021;18:613–22.

10. Wood KE. Major pulmonary embolism: review of a pathophysiologic approach to the golden hour of hemodynamically significant pulmonary embolism. Chest 2002;121:877–905.

11. Rosenberger P, Shernan SK, Shekar PS, et al. Acute hemodynamic collapse after induction of general anesthesia for emergent pulmonary embolectomy. Anesth Analg 2006;102:1311–5.

12. García-Cruz E, Manzur-Sandoval D, Baeza-Herrera LA, et al. Acute right ventricular failure in COVID-19 infection: a case series. J Cardiol Cases 2021;24:45–8.

13. Wilkinson-Stokes M. Right ventricular myocardial infarction and adverse events from nitrates: a narrative review. Australas J Paramed 2021;18.

14. Goldstein JA. Pathophysiology and management of right heart ischemia. J Am Coll Cardiol 2002;40:841–53.

15. Levin, T. & Goldstein, J. Right ventricular myocardial infarction. In: UpToDate, Post TW (Ed), UpToDate, Waltham, MA. (Accessed March 18, 2022)

16. Schouver ED, Chiche O, Bouvier P, et al. Diuretics versus volume expansion in acute submassive pulmonary embolism. Arch Cardiovasc Dis. 2017 Nov;110(11):616–625. Available at: https://www.sciencedirect.com/science/article/pii/S1875213617301651.

17. Jardin F, Gueret P, Prost JF, et al. Two-dimensional echocardiographic assessment of left ventricular function in chronic obstructive pulmonary disease. Am Rev Respir Dis 1984;129:135–42.

18. Belenkie I, Dani R, Smith ER, et al. Effects of volume loading during experimental acute pulmonary embolism. Circulation 1989;80:178–88.

19. Ventetuolo CE, Klinger JR. Management of acute right ventricular failure in the intensive care unit. Ann Am Thorac Soc 2014;11:811–22.

20. Olsson KM, Halank M, Egenlauf B, et al. Decompensated right heart failure, intensive care and perioperative management in patients with pulmonary hypertension: Updated recommendations from the Cologne Consensus Conference 2018. Int J Cardiol 2018;272S:46–52.

21. Hoeper MM, Benza RL, Corris P, et al. Intensive care, right ventricular support and lung transplantation in patients with pulmonary hypertension. Eur Respir J 2019;53:1801906.
22. Couture EJ, Tremblay J-A, Elmi-Sarabi M, et al. Noninvasive administration of inhaled epoprostenol and inhaled milrinone in extubated, spontaneously breathing patients with right ventricular failure and portal hypertension: a report of 2 cases. AA Pract 2019;12:208–11.
23. Yurtseven N, Karaca P, Uysal G, et al. A comparison of the acute hemodynamic effects of inhaled nitroglycerin and iloprost in patients with pulmonary hypertension undergoing mitral valve surgery. Ann Thorac Cardiovasc Surg 2006;12: 319–23.
24. Vahdatpour CA, Ryan JJ, Zimmerman JM, et al. Advanced airway management and respiratory care in decompensated pulmonary hypertension. Heart Fail Rev 2021. https://doi.org/10.1007/s10741-021-10168-9.

Evaluation and Management of Asthma and Chronic Obstructive Pulmonary Disease Exacerbation in the Emergency Department

Brit Long, MD[a],*, Salim R. Rezaie, MD[b],[1]

KEYWORDS

- Obstructive lung disease • Asthma • COPD • Acute exacerbation • Pulmonary

KEY POINTS

- Asthma and chronic obstructive pulmonary disease are obstructive airway diseases that can result in severe morbidity and mortality if not appropriately managed in the emergency department.
- History and examination are essential in diagnosing the condition, assessing exacerbation severity, and evaluating for mimics. Other evaluation adjuncts include chest radiograph, point-of-care ultrasound, capnography, and electrocardiogram.
- First-line treatments for acute exacerbation include bronchodilators and corticosteroids.
- Patients with severe exacerbation may benefit from intravenous magnesium, ketamine, and epinephrine. Noninvasive ventilation can also assist those with severe exacerbation.
- Mechanical ventilation is challenging and should use an obstructive lung strategy with permissive hypercapnia.

INTRODUCTION

Asthma and chronic obstructive pulmonary disease (COPD) are two obstructive pulmonary conditions that commonly require evaluation and management in the emergency department (ED) setting. More than 25 million Americans suffer from asthma, and asthma exacerbation is responsible for more than 2 million ED visits annually in the United States.[1–3] Asthma is more common in adult women as compared with men; however, in pediatric patients asthma affects men more than women. More

---

[a] SAUSHEC, Brooke Army Medical Center, Fort Sam Houston, TX, USA; [b] Emergency Medicine/Internal Medicine, Greater San Antonio Emergency Physcians (GSEP)
[1] Present address: 18014 Granite Hill Drive, San Antonio, TX 78255.
* Corresponding author. 317 Elmhurst Avenue, San Antonio, TX 78209.
E-mail address: brit.long@yahoo.com

Emerg Med Clin N Am 40 (2022) 539–563
https://doi.org/10.1016/j.emc.2022.05.007
0733-8627/22/Published by Elsevier Inc.

emed.theclinics.com

than 3500 patients die from asthma exacerbation every year.[1,4–6] Black Americans are three times more likely to die from asthma exacerbation as compared with White Americans, and adults are three times more likely to die than pediatric patients.[1,4,5] COPD affects more than 16 million adults in the United States and is the third global leading cause of death, with more than 1.5 million ED visits annually.[7–11] It accounts for close to 20% of all hospitalizations for patients over the age of 65 years.[9] These conditions are each associated with more than approximately $50 billion in health care expenditures every year, and unfortunately, visits and inpatient admissions for asthma and COPD exacerbation are increasing.[11,12]

Asthma and COPD are chronic diseases classically defined by airflow obstruction reversibility, but they differ regarding the specific component of the pulmonary system involved, prognosis, and local inflammation. It can also be difficult to differentiate them clinically in adults, and both conditions are associated with significant morbidity and mortality if not appropriately managed.[11,13–18] Thus, emergency clinicians must understand the acute evaluation and management of the patient with obstructive lung disease exacerbation.

DEFINITIONS

As discussed previously, asthma and COPD differ in several respects, including their definitions. The Global Initiative for Asthma defines asthma as an allergic disease that typically begins as a child.[14] It is marked by bronchial hyperresponsiveness, vascular permeability, bronchial smooth muscle spasm, and inflammatory mediator release.[6,8,14] Exacerbations are episodic and often vary in severity, most commonly presenting with coughing, wheezing, chest tightness, and shortness of breath.[14,15] There are a variety of triggers of acute exacerbations, including allergens, infection, emotional state, exercise, or exposure to an inhaled agent, but these exacerbations usually resolve completely with therapy or even spontaneously.[14,15]

COPD is defined by the Global Initiative for Chronic Obstructive Lung Disease as a preventable but acquired disease that most commonly results from tobacco smoking.[8,11] It is associated with persistent airflow obstruction with progressive decline in pulmonary function, with development in the fourth decade of life. Patients usually present with cough, sputum production, and shortness of breath.[11,13,16] Unlike asthma, COPD is associated with progressive airflow limitations and abnormal inflammatory response.[11,13,16]

PATHOPHYSIOLOGY

Although patients with asthma and COPD exacerbation present with similar symptoms, the primary difference between them is the inflammatory cells that cause airway obstruction. In asthma, eosinophils, mast cells, and CD4 cells are the primary mediators, resulting in airway hyperresponsiveness and narrowing, mucous plugging, hyperinflation, atelectasis, and ventilation/perfusion mismatch.[6,14,15] In COPD, neutrophils, macrophages, and CD8 cells result in inflammation.[7,8,13] This results in small airway narrowing and reduction in alveoli with increased mucous production. Owing to the specific cells involved, asthma is more rapidly reversible with corticosteroids, whereas COPD is associated with progressive damage to the pulmonary system and a decline in respiratory function (**Table 1**).[6–8,13–15] Owing to the underlying pathophysiology, patients with severe asthma or COPD exacerbation can present with severe bronchospasm and obstruction, and in later stages, patients may present with significant respiratory fatigue leading to hypercapnia and hypoxemia.

Table 1
Asthma and chronic obstructive pulmonary disease differences

Component	Asthma	COPD
Cells	CD4 cells, mast cells, and eosinophils	CD8 cells, macrophages, and neutrophils
Site affected	Proximal airways (peripheral airways in severe exacerbation)	Peripheral airway, lung parenchyma, and pulmonary vessels
Airway obstruction	Reversible: bronchoconstriction, mucous edema, and mucous plugs	Not fully reversible: small airway fibrosis, emphysema, mucous exudates, and mucous edema
Etiology	Allergens, cold, exercise, and so forth	Tobacco use and pulmonary irritant
Age of first symptoms	Usually childhood/younger age	Over 40 y
Course	Variable exacerbations, remission, can be progressive	Progressive decline with exacerbations
Bronchodilator response	Positive	Moderate to poor
Corticosteroid response	Positive	Moderate to poor

INITIAL EMERGENCY DEPARTMENT EVALUATION

The emergency clinician must perform a methodical but focused history and physical examination in patients with obstructive lung disease, as there are many conditions that may initially present with dyspnea and mimic asthma or COPD (**Box 1**, **Fig. 1**). In critically ill patients presenting with severe respiratory distress, history may be limited, but, if able, should include time of symptom onset, etiology/underlying cause, presence of systemic symptoms (ie, fevers, chills, rigors), attempted treatments before arrival, and prior care for the disease.[11,14–20] Historical factors such as recent ED visits or hospital admissions for obstructive lung disease, increased use of short-acting beta-agonist (SABA) therapy, recent steroid use, recent antibiotic use, previous airway interventions (noninvasive ventilation [NIV], endotracheal intubation), and prior intensive care unit (ICU) admission are associated with uncontrolled disease and greater risk of severe exacerbation.[11,14–20] Patients typically present with cough, wheezing, dyspnea, and chest tightness. Patients with the inability to speak more than a few words, agitation, respiratory distress, and air hunger reflect a severe exacerbation.[11,14–16] Physical examination should focus on cardiorespiratory status; vital signs; and the presence of air movement, fevers, wheezing, cyanosis, and altered mental status.[15–18] Evidence of severe exacerbation includes tachypnea, tachycardia, use of accessory muscles, speaking one to two words at a time, tripod position, and inability to lie flat (see **Fig. 1**). However, the absence of these findings should not be used to exclude severe exacerbation (ie, a lack of wheezing that can indicate severe obstruction).[11,14,15] Signs suggesting cardiorespiratory distress and imminent arrest include bradycardia, cyanosis, decreased mental status, and inability to maintain respiratory effort.[15,16]

DIAGNOSIS
Laboratory Evaluation

No laboratory test exists that can identify obstructive airway disease exacerbation as the cause of dyspnea. However, laboratory assessment may assist in evaluating for other causes, such as heart failure and cardiac ischemia. Significant elevation of brain natriuretic peptide suggests heart failure, and troponin may be used to assess for non-ST elevation myocardial infarction.[15,16,21,22] D-dimer can be used in appropriately selected patients in evaluation for pulmonary embolism (PE).[23,24] Complete blood count may reveal anemia or leukocytosis, whereas a comprehensive metabolic panel may reveal renal injury or electrolyte abnormalities. C-reactive protein (CRP) has been suggested as one determinant of the need for antibiotics in those with acute exacerbation of COPD.[11,25] Sputum samples are not recommended in the ED, as they are unreliable and do not affect ED management unless the clinician suspects tuberculosis.[11,16] Viral testing may assist for the evaluation of an underlying etiology, including COVID-19 and influenza.[16,26,27]

Blood Gas

Several guidelines include blood gas assessment in the evaluation of patients with asthma and COPD exacerbation. Arterial blood gas (ABG) can evaluate partial pressure of carbon dioxide (P_{CO_2}) and partial pressure of oxygen.[15,16,28] Although the ABG may be used in those with severe patients requiring respiratory support, mechanical ventilation, or those who fail initial therapies, ABG is no longer a routine test performed in the ED to evaluate the severity of asthma or COPD exacerbation, as ABG is associated with several significant risk factors such as aneurysm formation, arterial injury, infection, and even loss of limb. However, venous blood gas (VBG) is not associated with these complications and can assist in evaluating a patient respiratory status.[14–16,28–35] Early in the exacerbation, VBG will reveal low P_{CO_2} due to tachypnea, but as the exacerbation continues, the P_{CO_2} can begin to increase because of worsening obstruction and poor ventilation. VBG is an effective, reliable screening tool for hypercarbia, as P_{CO_2} less than 45 mm Hg can exclude hypercarbia.[29–31,33,35] Importantly, blood gas assessment cannot accurately predict the need for intubation

---

Box 1
Common mimics of asthma and chronic obstructive pulmonary disease

Acute bronchopulmonary aspergillosis

Anaphylaxis

Angioedema

Central airway obstruction

Congestive heart failure

Drug reaction

Eosinophilic granulomatosis with polyangiitis

Foreign body aspiration

Gastroesophageal reflux disease

Hypersensitivity pneumonitis

Pneumonia

Pulmonary ascariasis

Pulmonary embolism

Vocal cord dysfunction

Upper respiratory infection

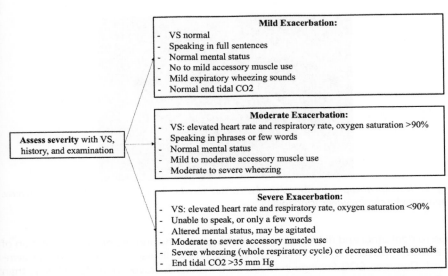

Mild Exacerbation:
- VS normal
- Speaking in full sentences
- Normal mental status
- No to mild accessory muscle use
- Mild expiratory wheezing sounds
- Normal end tidal CO2

Moderate Exacerbation:
- VS: elevated heart rate and respiratory rate, oxygen saturation >90%
- Speaking in phrases or few words
- Normal mental status
- Mild to moderate accessory muscle use
- Moderate to severe wheezing

Assess severity with VS, history, and examination

Severe Exacerbation:
- VS: elevated heart rate and respiratory rate, oxygen saturation <90%
- Unable to speak, or only a few words
- Altered mental status, may be agitated
- Moderate to severe accessory muscle use
- Severe wheezing (whole respiratory cycle) or decreased breath sounds
- End tidal CO2 >35 mm Hg

Fig. 1. Airway obstructive disease severity. CO2, carbon dioxide; g, grams; IV, intravenous; mm Hg, millimeters mercury; VS, vital signs.

or the risk of mortality.[11,15,28–35] Clinical examination should remain the focus. In patients who fail to respond to initial therapies, visible respiratory distress/fatigue, or evidence of hypercarbia (ie, altered mental status, somnolence), a blood gas can assist in evaluating for hypercarbia and ventilation/perfusion mismatch.[11,15,28–35] Clinicians can also use trends in P_{CO_2} and clinical assessment to evaluate treatment response.

Capnography

Capnography can be useful in risk stratifying patients with acute exacerbation. In the initial stages, patients may be tachypneic and result in lower end-tidal CO_2 ($EtCO_2$) levels, but in those with severe exacerbation, an elevated EtCO2 suggests hypercarbia.[36–38] Increased EtCO2 is correlated with the dead space volume to tidal volume ratio. Airway obstruction from bronchospasm can result in an increased slope of phase 3 with an increased alpha angle similar to a shark fin (**Fig. 2**).[38] Studies suggest that beta-agonist therapy can decrease the slope of phase 3, reflecting improved air movement and respiratory status.[38–42]

Spirometry

Several guidelines, including Global Initiative for Asthma (GINA) and Global Initiative for Chronic Obstructive Pulmonary Disease (GOLD), recommend spirometry to assist in diagnosis, classification, and treatment of obstructive airway disease.[11,14–16] However, performing spirometry in the ED setting is not recommended, especially in the undifferentiated patient with dyspnea. Patients with severe exacerbation are unlikely to be able to perform the necessary peak flow measurement due to the effort required.[15–18]

Electrocardiogram

Electrocardiogram (ECG) is an integral test for patients who present with dyspnea. In COPD, acute cardiovascular events are a significant cause of death, which may be due to dysrhythmias.[43–47] These are predominantly present in patients with COPD

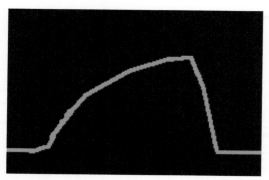

Fig. 2. Waveform capnography with obstructive airway disease. (*Image from* http://www. capnography.com/new/encyclopedia.)

due to right atrial and right ventricular (RV) hypertrophy and the clockwise rotation of the heart. P waves may become more vertical due to displacement of the heart downward. Common ECG findings in COPD also include S waves in leads I–III; less than 1 R/s ratio in leads V5 or V6; isoelectric P wave, QRS amplitude less than 1.5 mm, T wave amplitude less than 0.5 mm in lead I; P wave in lead aVL; or P wave amplitude in lead III > lead I. The most common dysrhythmias in patients with COPD include atrial fibrillation/flutter and multifocal atrial tachycardia.[43–49]

Radiography

Chest radiograph is a common imaging modality obtained in patients with acute dyspnea. Patients with obstructive lung disease often show an increased anteroposterior diameter, flattened diaphragm, enlarged retrosternal airspace, bullae, and narrow vertical cardiac silhouette (**Fig. 3**).[16,50–53] Although chest radiograph has poor sensitivity in acute COPD exacerbation, studies reveal that chest radiograph affects management in more than 20% of cases.[51] Another retrospective analysis found that 84% of chest radiographs contributed to the evaluation and management of patients with COPD.[53] Chest radiographs are recommended in patients with COPD exacerbation to evaluate for other causes of shortness of breath including pneumonia, pulmonary edema, and pneumothorax. In patients with asthma, chest radiograph is more controversial and requires clinical judgment.[14,15] Although it is not recommended on a routine basis in those with asthma, it should be considered in patients with evidence of another condition such as pneumonia (ie, fever), those in extremis, patients not responding to initial therapies, those at risk of a different diagnosis (ie, heart failure or foreign body aspiration), and patients with new-onset wheezing or a new diagnosis of obstructive lung disease.[15–18]

Ultrasound

Point-of-care ultrasound (POCUS) is an integral tool in the ED setting. It is rapid, reliable, and not associated with radiation exposure. POCUS can be an adjunct in determining the underlying cause of the patient's dyspnea (**Fig. 4**). Hepatized lung tissue or B-lines suggest pulmonary edema (**Fig. 5**).[54–58] Evaluation of the heart may reveal a distended RV (**Fig. 6**), pericardial effusion that may suggest cardiac tamponade (**Fig. 7**), or poor ejection fraction. The absence of lung sliding suggests pneumothorax (**Fig. 8**). Several imaging protocols include the bedside lung ultrasonography in emergency, fluid administration limited by lung sonography, and lung ultrasound in the

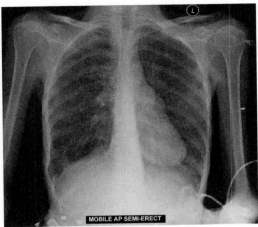

Fig. 3. Chest radiograph with severe emphysema and lung hyperexpansion. (*Obtained from* https://radiopaedia.org/cases/severe-copd-and-pectus-excavatum?lang=us. *Case courtesy of* Dr Henry Knipe, Radiopaedia.org, rID: 39471.)

critically ill.[54–58] A study published in 2013 found ultrasound improved accuracy in diagnosing pneumonia, COPD, heart failure, and PE.[58] Another trial found POCUS was 95% accurate in diagnosing COPD or asthma exacerbation, with an overall accuracy of 90% for determining the etiology of dyspnea.[57]

MANAGEMENT

Management is based on the severity of exacerbation and should occur concurrently with ED evaluation, particularly in those with severe exacerbation (**Fig. 9**).[15,16]

Oxygen Supplementation

Oxygen is a key component in managing the hypoxic patient with dyspnea. Hypoxia in patients with acute asthma exacerbation should be immediately addressed with oxygen supplementation[14,15,59–62]; however, in patients with acute COPD exacerbation, guidelines recommend maintaining oxygen levels between 88% and 92%.[11,16] In patients with acute COPD exacerbation, bronchodilators should be administered with compressed air, not oxygen. This titrated oxygen approach in those with COPD is associated with reduced mortality.[16,63–65] For patients with acute COPD exacerbation and with oxygen saturation greater than 92%, no further supplementation is needed. In those with saturations between 85% and 92%, oxygen at 2 to 3 L/min with nasal cannula can be used, whereas for those with a saturation less than 85%, a face mask or Venturi mask with high flows can be used.[16,63–66]

Bronchodilators

Bronchodilators are the first-line medication used in patients with obstructive lung disease, as they treat bronchial hyperreactivity and can reduce or even reverse airflow obstruction in both asthma and acute exacerbation of COPD (AECOPD).[15,16,66] Bronchodilators include short-acting beta-2 agonists and ipratropium bromide. Of note, the method of delivery may include a metered-dose inhaler or gas-driven nebulizer. Current evidence does not show a difference in patient-centered outcomes between the two routes.[15,67,68] However, in those with severe exacerbation, nebulized therapy

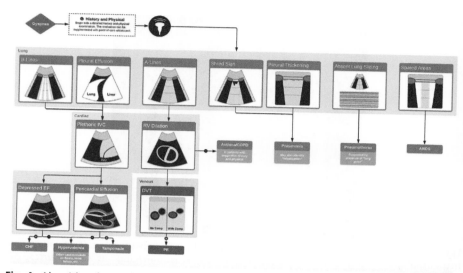

Fig. 4. Algorithm for evaluation of dyspnea using POCUS. Courtesy of Dr. Tom Fadial, MD.

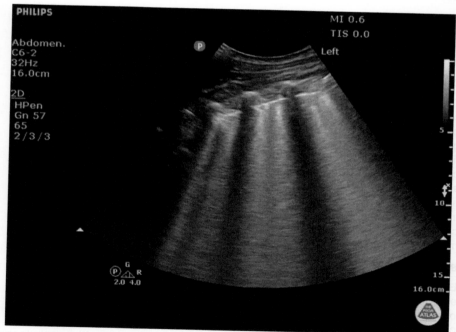

Fig. 5. Multiple B lines suggestive of pulmonary edema. (*Obtained from* the Pocus Atlas at https://www.thepocusatlas.com/new-blog/2018/3/14/ddxof-pocus-for-undifferentiated-shortness-of-breath.)

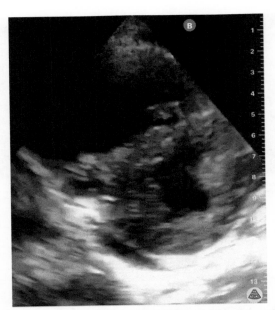

Fig. 6. Distended RV. (*Obtained from* the Pocus Atlas at https://www.thepocusatlas.com/new-blog/2018/3/14/ddxof-pocus-for-undifferentiated-shortness-of-breath.)

is recommended due to the cooperation needed for proper metered dose inhaler (MDI) administration.

SABAs stimulate airway beta-2 receptors, which increases intracellular cyclic adenosine monophosphate, ultimately resulting in pulmonary smooth muscle relaxation.

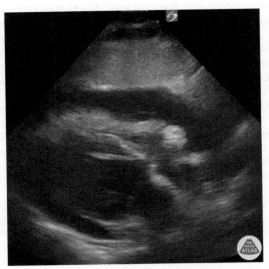

Fig. 7. Pericardial effusion with evidence of tamponade. (*Obtained from* the Pocus Atlas at https://www.thepocusatlas.com/new-blog/2018/3/14/ddxof-pocus-for-undifferentiated-shortness-of-breath.)

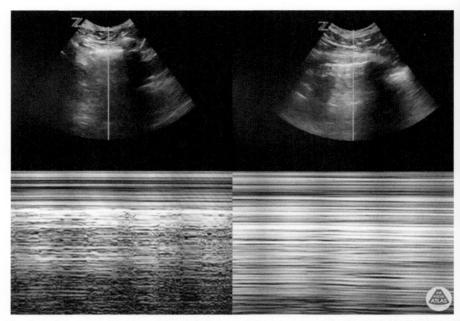

Fig. 8. Left image with normal lung sliding and right image with absent lung sliding in a patient with pneumothorax. (*Obtained from* the Pocus Atlas at https://www.thepocusatlas.com/new-blog/2018/3/14/ddxof-pocus-for-undifferentiated-shortness-of-breath.)

The time of onset is usually within seconds to minutes. The peak effect approaches 30 min, with a half-life of 4 to 6 h.[11,14–16] Albuterol is the most common SABA used in the ED, consisting of an R and S enantiomer. The R enantiomer is the active form that results in bronchodilation, and the S enantiomer is thought to cause tremors, tachycardia, and anxiety.[15,69] However, studies of levalbuterol, which consists of the purified R enantiomer, do not show superiority over nebulized albuterol or improvement in safety.[68,70–72] In those with severe asthma exacerbation, continuous nebulized albuterol at a dose of 10 to 20 mg per hour is recommended, with a number needed to treat (NNT) to reduce hospitalization of 10.[15,73]

Long-acting beta-2 agonists (LABAs) include salmeterol and formoterol to provide close to 12 h of bronchodilation, but evidence suggests increased exacerbations and mortality when used in asthma patients.[74–78] In COPD, LABAs can improve lung function and quality of life and reduce exacerbation severity and frequency.[74–80] LABAs are typically combined with an inhaled corticosteroid for therapy, and these can be considered for patients as a discharge prescription for maintenance therapy.[79,81]

Inhaled epinephrine may assist patients who have not improved with other SABA agents due to its alpha activity reducing airway edema, but current evidence has not shown improved efficacy in comparison with SABA therapy.[82–86]

Anticholinergics

Ipratropium bromide when inhaled competitively inhibits muscarinic acetylcholine receptors in the pulmonary smooth muscle, resulting in bronchodilation. When

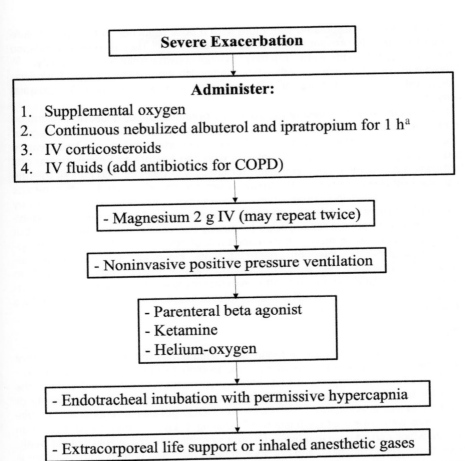

Fig. 9. Management of severe obstructive disease. [a]May repeat albuterol multiple times if no improvement after first hour.

compared with SABAs, ipratropium is slower in onset but lasts longer.[14,15,18] The time of onset approximates 15 min, and the peak effect is 60 to 90 min with a half-life of 6 to 8 h.[15,87] Use of ipratropium has been associated with reduced exacerbations, hospital admission, and length of stay in asthma, with an NNT of 1 to reduce hospitalization in acute asthma.[88–93] Although GOLD guidelines recommend using a SABA first in AECOPD, the literature suggests combing albuterol with ipratropium is more effective in bronchodilation and reducing hospital admission.[11,92] Ipratropium is administered in doses of 0.5 to 2 mg for the first hour. Tiotropium is a longer acting anticholinergic often used for maintenance therapy in those with COPD and can improve symptom control in those on an inhaled corticosteroid and LABA, or if used alone.[94,95]

Corticosteroids

Corticosteroids are an integral therapy in patients with an obstructive airway exacerbation, as they upregulate beta receptors and reduce airway inflammation.[11,14–18] Current guidelines recommend corticosteroids in those with moderate or severe exacerbation and those who do not initially respond to SABA therapy.[11,14,18,96–98]

Corticosteroids are associated with more than a 50% reduction in treatment failure and an NNT of 9 to prevent one treatment failure.[15,96–98] They also reduce relapse rates and hospital length of stay, but they have not shown a reduction in mortality.[15,98] Although the onset of action is within 6 h of administration, studies suggest administration within the first hour of ED care may reduce the need for hospital admission.[15,16,96–98]

There is currently controversy regarding the optimal steroid, dose, administration route, and treatment duration.[15,16] Oral and parenteral corticosteroids show similar bioavailability and patient outcomes, although oral corticosteroids are less invasive and less expensive.[15,16] Thus, for patients who can tolerate oral medications, oral formulation is recommended. However, for critically ill patients who cannot tolerate oral administration, parenteral treatment is recommended. Inhaled corticosteroids administered with inhaled albuterol can improve smooth muscle relaxation and airway function.[81,99] There is no benefit with doses over prednisone 2 mg/kg per day or equivalent including treatment failure, need for airway intervention, or length of stay, but higher doses are associated with increased risk of adverse events including myopathy, hyperglycemia, infection, gastrointestinal bleeding, and neurologic effects.[100–104] Literature has evaluated the duration of therapy ranging from 5 to 8 days. The REDUCE trial found shorter term therapy was non-inferior to longer duration with no difference in mortality, relapse rate, or lung function recovery, and 5 days of treatment is recommended at this time.[105]

Magnesium

Intravenous (IV) administration of magnesium sulfate may result in calcium receptor blockade or activation of adenylyl cyclase, leading to pulmonary smooth relaxation.[15,18] Literature suggests it may improve pulmonary function and reduce the need for hospital admission by 25%, but data do not show reduced mortality or need for airway intervention.[106–109] GINA and GOLD guidelines recommend its use in patients with severe exacerbations.[11,14] Dosing is 2g IV administered more than 20 min, which can be repeated twice. Of note, possible adverse events include weakness, hypotension, flushing, and changes in heart rate, and IV fluid administration is recommended with the administration of magnesium. Inhaled administration is controversial, with literature to date demonstrating no benefit.[110,111]

Ketamine

Ketamine is a dissociative analgesic that may be used in patients who are refractory to other therapies. It has a rapid onset of action within 60 seconds and a distribution of 7 to 11 min.[15,16,112] Ketamine is an N-methyl-D-aspartic acid receptor antagonist in the lung parenchyma, which can reduce pulmonary edema and bronchoconstriction.[113] It can also reduce the production of nitric oxide, which reduces bronchospasm.[114] Finally, ketamine blocks recruitment of macrophages and reduces cytokine production.[112–114] Ultimately, ketamine can reduce airway hyperinflammation and hyperreactivity, whereas decreased bronchospasm, with studies finding improved pulmonary function, reduced oxygen requirement, and decreased requirement for invasive ventilation.[112–116] However, as ketamine has analgesic, anesthetic, and amnestic qualities, it should be administered in a monitored environment.[112,115] It can be administered using two dosing strategies. Sub-dissociative dose ketamine (0.05–0.4 mg/kg/h) is used to reduce bronchospasm and improve pulmonary function while not sedating the patient, and dissociative dosed ketamine (0.5–2.0 mg/kg) can be used for delayed sequence intubation or induction for rapid sequence intubation.[112–116] Ketamine can also increase bronchial secretions and relieve mucous plugs.[112–116]

Parenteral Beta Agonist Therapy

Parenteral beta-agonists are usually reserved for patients with severe exacerbation who do not respond to other therapies. Terbutaline was previously a common parenteral beta-agonist therapy administered via the subcutaneous (SC) route.[14,15] However, data do not show an improvement in those with severe exacerbation who are unresponsive to other therapies.[14,15] In patients with severe exacerbation or anaphylaxis, epinephrine 0.3 to 0.5 mg intramuscular (IM) may be administered. The IM route is recommended over the SC route, as patients with cardiorespiratory distress or failure have a hyperadrenergic state with reduced skin circulation.[15] For patients refractory to IM dosing or those who are profoundly hypotensive, epinephrine should be administered via the IV route in doses of 5 to 20 μg every 2 to 5 min, or via infusion 0.1 to 0.5 mcg/kg/min[15,117] Parenteral epinephrine may result in anxiety, nausea, and tremor, but most patients have no adverse events from IV epinephrine. Literature suggests that vital signs, including heart rate, blood pressure, and respiratory rate, normalize in those receiving parenteral epinephrine due to reduced bronchospasm.[15,16,117–119]

Heliox

Heliox is a mixture of helium and oxygen that can reduce airflow turbulence through narrow airways. It may also improve ventilation/perfusion matching and improve the elimination of carbon dioxide.[120,121] Studies suggest that heliox-driven bronchodilation can provide faster and larger increases in forced expiratory volume, forced vital capacity, and expiratory flow rate, with reduced ED admissions.[121,122] If used, it should be considered as an adjunct early in the patient course before increased oxygen requirements.

Antibiotics

Antibiotics are not recommended in patients with acute asthma exacerbation with no evidence of underlying bacterial infection. However, antibiotics are a central component of acute COPD exacerbation management in those with increased dyspnea, purulent sputum, or increased sputum production.[11,16,123] We also recommend antibiotics in patients with severe symptoms requiring hospitalization or airway intervention. Antibiotics in those with COPD exacerbation are associated with an NNT of 3 to prevent conservative treatment failure and 8 to prevent short-term mortality.[11,16,123] Pulmonary infection is the precipitant of more than 80% of patients with acute COPD exacerbation, with half of these due to bacterial infection, although this is not the case in patients with asthma exacerbation.[124–126] Antibiotic therapy in those with acute COPD exacerbation is associated with reduced risk of progressing to pneumonia, decreased pulmonary inflammation, and improved bacterial eradication.[127] Antibiotics should be chosen based on local susceptibility patterns and history of recent antibiotic use. For those who have received antibiotics in the last 3 months, an alternative antibiotic class should be used.[16,128] For discharged patients who are otherwise well but meet the criteria for antibiotics, azithromycin, doxycycline, or levofloxacin should be used.[16,128] For patients who are unhealthy, levofloxacin, moxifloxacin, or amoxicillin/clavulanate are recommended. Patients who will be admitted should receive levofloxacin, cefepime, ceftazidime, or piperacillin/tazobactam if *Pseudomonas* is a suspected cause, whereas levofloxacin, moxifloxacin, ceftriaxone, or cefotaxime may be used if the patient does not have risk factors for *Pseudomonas*.[16,128] CRP has shown promise in determining the need for antibiotics, with one study of patients with mild-to-moderate exacerbation showed that patients with CRP less than 40 mg/L were less likely to benefit from antibiotics.[25] Other patients with COPD and mild symptoms can be managed as an outpatient without antibiotics.[11,16] If influenza is the underlying etiology of exacerbation, oseltamivir can be used.[16,129]

Noninvasive Ventilation

Bilevel positive airway pressure/continuous positive airway pressure

Airway management of the patient with obstructive lung disease can be challenging. Early recognition and management of patients with severe exacerbation can prevent further patient decompensation and improve survival.[15,16] NIV with a full face mask is a vital component of therapy in the patient with severe exacerbation. NIV can function as a direct bronchodilator and recruit alveoli through positive end-expiratory pressure, which improves ventilation/perfusion mismatching and reduces work of breathing.[15,16,130–135] Evidence suggests NIV can reduce hospital admission rates, ICU length of stay, overall hospital length of stay, and mortality in patients with acute COPD exacerbation.[15,16,133–135] Although early literature regarding the use of NIV in severe asthma exacerbation did not show clear benefits,[15,16,133–135] several recent retrospective studies have found NIV to be safe and effective, reducing the risk of mortality and the need for invasive mechanical ventilation.[136,137] Absolute contraindications include cardiac or respiratory arrest, whereas relative contraindications include the patient who is uncooperative, has copious secretions, and has a deformity of the face or upper airway and recent esophageal trauma or surgery.[15,16] Of note, altered mental status, pH < 7.25, and hypercarbia are not contraindications if the clinician can closely monitor the patient. NIV can improve mental status in patients with hypercarbia, as NIV improves ventilation.[15,131,138] The clinician must closely monitor the patient on NIV, evaluating the work of breathing and modifying settings based on patient response. Bilevel positive airway pressure provides an inspiratory pressure and expiratory pressure, which likely is more beneficial compared with continuous positive airway pressure in obstructive lung disease, which is a problem with ventilation. Initial settings should include an inspiratory pressure support of 5 to 10 mm Hg and PEEP of 3 to 5 mm Hg.[15,16,133] If titrating, the inspiratory pressure should be increased while maintaining PEEP. Maximal medical management should be continued while the patient is on NIV, including inline, inhaled bronchodilator therapy.

High-flow nasal cannula

A high-flow nasal cannula (HFNC) is a relatively newer device that provides heated and humidified oxygen via nasal cannula with a flow rate of up 60 L/min[15,139,140] This modality can be beneficial in patients who are unable to tolerate a face mask or with contraindications to NIV. Although HFNC reduces anatomic dead space, increases airway pressure, and decreases resistance to expiratory flow, it does not actively improve tidal volume.[15,139–144] Compared with facemask NIV, HFNC may improve thoracoabdominal synchrony, and the HFNC delivered oxygen flows better reflect the predicted fraction of inspired oxygen.[140,142–144]

Endotracheal Intubation

Endotracheal intubation and mechanical ventilation are reserved for those with progressing respiratory distress who fail typical therapies and NIV, respiratory or cardiac arrest, and altered mental status/coma.[15,16,145–147] However, the decision to intubate is difficult, as airway manipulation may worsen bronchospasm and result in laryngospasm. Mortality rates reach 20% in patients intubated with obstructive lung disease.[146]

Patients with obstructive lung disease undergoing endotracheal intubation should be considered a difficult airway, with the most experienced operator performing the procedure.[15,16] Maximal preoxygenation and rapid sequence intubation are recommended. Induction agents such as ketamine or propofol may be used.[148,149] Ketamine is an optimal induction agent (1–2 mg/kg IV), as it relaxes bronchial smooth muscle and has analgesic and sedative properties, although it may result in hypertension and arrhythmias due to catecholamine release.[112–114,150] Propofol possesses some bronchodilating effects but can result in hypotension.[150] Although sedation-only intubation is possible, we recommend using a paralytic to improve first-pass success. Rocuronium at a dose of 1.2 mg/kg IV has equivalent time to onset compared with succinylcholine, although rocuronium does have a longer duration of action, especially with higher doses.[151] Succinylcholine side effects include bradycardia, hyperkalemia, fasciculations, and malignant hyperthermia, whereas rocuronium can cause anaphylaxis.[151]

Before intubation, patient hemodynamics should be optimized. A fluid bolus can improve preload. This is especially important when the patient is placed on mechanical ventilation, which abruptly increases intrathoracic pressure and decreases venous return.[138,146] A vasopressor such as norepinephrine is also recommended if the patient is hypotensive.

Mechanical Ventilation

Following endotracheal intubation and tube securement and confirmation, clinicians must use mechanical ventilation settings to prevent hyperinflation and auto-PEEP, which result in hemodynamic collapse and barotrauma.[135,138,152] Ventilator settings with a reduced respiratory rate and tidal volume shorten inspiratory time and lengthen exhalation, resulting in permissive hypercapnia.[138,146] Initial settings should include volume control with a respiratory rate of 6 to 10 breaths per minute, tidal volume 6-8 cc/kg ideal body weight, and inspiratory flow rate 80 to 120 L/min[138,146] An inspiration-to-expiration ratio of greater than 1:4 is also recommended, which increases expiratory time.[138,146] Patients also require scheduled inline, inhaled

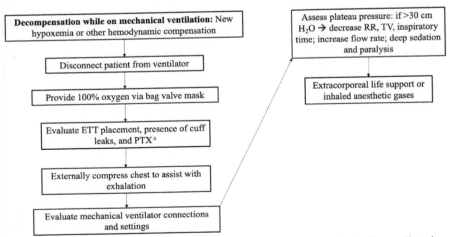

Fig. 10. Evaluation and management of the decompensating mechanically ventilated patient. cm H_2O, centimeters of water; ETT, endotracheal tube; PTX, pneumothorax; RR, respiratory rate; TV, tidal volume. [a]Can evaluate ETT placement and for pneumothorax with ultrasound.

bronchodilator therapy. Metered-dose inhalers may reduce the risk of nosocomial pneumonia compared with nebulization.[153] Deep sedation is also recommended to improve patient lung mechanics. Although prolonged paralysis can be used to improve patient–ventilator compliance, it is not recommended due to the increased risk of pneumonia and ICU length of stay.[154] Decompensation while on the ventilator requires consideration of several factors, as shown in **Fig. 10**.

Extracorporeal Membrane Oxygenation

Extracorporeal membrane oxygenation (ECMO) is a final option in treatment-refractory patients. ECMO can be considered in patients on mechanical ventilation with inadequate oxygenation or acidosis. It may be beneficial in those with pulmonary hyperinflation with reduced cardiac preload and output.[15,155] One study found ECMO improved airway exchange and oxygenation while mechanically ventilated, with 83.5% of patients surviving to discharge. However, more than 65% of patients experienced a complication such as hemorrhage.[155] ECMO also requires significant resources and support staff present in select centers.

Care Plans

Detailed asthma or COPD care plans are integral to patient care and improved outcomes. These plans typically include explicit discharge instruction, medications, and instructions on how to use them, self-assessment, action plan for managing recurrent obstruction, and follow-up appointment. These care plans are associated with medication compliance and improved patient outcomes.[11,14,79] Admitted patients on discharge should follow-up within 1 week. Pulmonary rehabilitation for those with COPD can prevent recurrent exacerbation.[79]

CLINICS CARE POINTS

- Patients with severe asthma or chronic obstructive pulmonary disease exacerbation can present with significant bronchospasm and obstruction. Patients can also present with respiratory fatigue leading to hypercapnia and hypoxemia.

- Adjunctive evaluation tools include capnography and ultrasound. These can assist in evaluating for other causes of dyspnea (eg, ultrasound for cardiac tamponade, pulmonary edema, and pneumothorax), and they can also be used to assess disease severity.

- Inhaled bronchodilators and intravenous corticosteroids are essential components of therapy. If patients do not respond to these measures, noninvasive ventilation (NIV) should be attempted with inline inhaled beta-agonists. Intravenous epinephrine and ketamine can also be used.

- Mechanical ventilation does not correct the underlying bronchospasm, but patients with respiratory failure and those who fail NIV should be intubated.

- If mechanically ventilated, permissive hypercapnia using ventilator settings that reduce respiratory rate and tidal volume with increased expiratory time is recommended. Adequate sedation is also necessary.

- If patients decompensate while mechanically ventilated, a structured approach for assessment and management is necessary.

- Extracorporeal membrane oxygenation can be considered for treatment-refractory patients.

DISCLOSURE

The authors have nothing to disclose.

REFERENCES

1. Centers for Disease Control and Prevention. 2019 national health interview survey data. U.S. Department of Health & Human Services; 2020. Available at: https://www.cdc.gov/asthma/nhis/2019/data.htm.
2. Moorman JE, Akinbami LJ, Bailey CM, et al. National surveillance of asthma:-United States, 2001–2010. National Center for Health Statistics. Vital Health Stat 3 2012;(35):1–58.
3. Akinbami LJ, Moorman JE, Liu X. Asthma prevalence, health care use, and mortality: United States, 2005-2009. Natl Health Stat Rep 2011;(32):1–14.
4. National Center for Health Statistics. National hospital Ambulatory medical care survey (2010-2018). U.S. Department of Health and Human Services, Centers for Disease Control and Prevention; 2019. Available at: https://www.cdc.gov/asthma/national-surveillance-data/healthcare-use.htm.
5. National Center for Health Statistics. National Vital Statistics System: Mortality (1999-2018). U.S. Department of Health and Human Services, Centers for Disease Control and Prevention. Available at: https://wonder.cdc.gov/ucd-icd10.html. Accessed September 1, 2021.
6. WHO. Asthma. Available at: https://www.who.int/news-room/fact-sheets/detail/asthma. Accessed September 1, 2021.
7. WHO. COPD. Available at: https://www.who.int/news-room/fact-sheets/detail/chronic-obstructive-pulmonary-disease-(copd). Accessed September 1, 2021.
8. Papaiwannou A, Zarogoulidis P, Porpodis K, et al. Asthma-chronic obstructive pulmonary disease overlap syndrome (ACOS): current literature review. J Thorac Dis 2014;6(Suppl 1):S146–51.
9. Mannino DM, Watt G, Hole D, et al. The natural history of chronic obstructive pulmonary disease. Eur Respir J 2006;27(3):627–43.
10. American Lung Association. Chronic obstructive pulmonary disease (COPD) fact sheet. Available at: http://www.lung.org/lung-disease/copd/resources/factsfigures/COPD-Fact-Sheet.html. Accessed November 24, 2014.
11. Global Initiative for Chronic Obstructive Lung Disease (GOLD). GOLD 2020 guidelines. Available at: https://goldcopd.org/. Accessed May 16, 2020.
12. CDC's Asthma's Impact on the Nation. Available at: http://www.cdc.gov/asthma/most_recent_data.htm. Accessed September 1, 2021.
13. Postma DS, Reddel HK, ten Hacken NH, et al. Asthma and chronic obstructive pulmonary disease: similarities and differences. Clin Chest Med 2014;35(1):143–56.
14. Global Initiative for Asthma (GINA). Global strategies for asthma management and prevention. 2015. Available at: www.ginasthma.org. Accessed September 1, 2021.
15. Long B, Lentz S, Koyfman A, et al. Evaluation and management of the critically ill adult asthmatic in the emergency department setting. Am J Emerg Med 2021;44:441–51.
16. Sorge R, DeBlieux P. Acute Exacerbations of Chronic Obstructive Pulmonary Disease: A Primer for Emergency Physicians. J Emerg Med 2020;59(5):643–59.
17. McFadden ER Jr. Acute severe asthma. Am J Respir Crit Care Med 2003;168(7):740–59.
18. Rodrigo GL. Advances in acute asthma. Curr Opin Pulm Med 2015;21(1):22–6.
19. Patel M, Pilcher J, Munro C, et al. Short-acting β-agonist use as a marker of current asthma control. J Allergy Clin Immunol Pract 2013;1(4):370–7.

20. Stanford RH, Shah MB, D'Souza AO, et al. Short-acting β-agonist use and its ability to predict future asthma-related outcomes. Ann Allergy Asthma Immunol 2012;109(6):403–7.

21. Kakouros NS, Kakouros SN. Clinical assessment in acute heart failure. Hellenic J Cardiol 2015;56:285–301.

22. Long B, Koyfman A, Gottlieb M. Diagnosis of Acute Heart Failure in the Emergency Department: An Evidence-Based Review. West J Emerg Med 2019; 20(6):875–84.

23. Coccia CB, Palkowski GH, Schweitzer B, et al. Dyspnoea: pathophysiology and a clinical approach. S Afr Med J 2016;106:32–6.

24. American College of Emergency Physicians Clinical Policies Subcommittee (Writing Committee) on Thromboembolic Disease, Wolf SJ, Hahn SA, Nentwich LM, et al. Clinical Policy: Critical Issues in the Evaluation and Management of Adult Patients Presenting to the Emergency Department With Suspected Acute Venous Thromboembolic Disease. Ann Emerg Med 2018;71(5): e59–109.

25. Miravitlles M, Moragas A, Hernandez S, et al. Is it possible to identify exacerbations of mild to moderate COPD that do not require antibiotic treatment? Chest 2013;144(5):1571–7.

26. Mohan A, Chandra S, Agarwal D, et al. Prevalence of viral infection detected by PCR and RT-PCR in patients with acute exacerbation of COPD: a systematic review. Respirology 2010;15(3):536–42.

27. Wu X, Chen D, Gu X, et al. Prevalence and risk of viral infection in patients with acute exacerbation of chronic obstructive pulmonary disease: a meta-analysis. Mol Biol Rep 2014;41(7):4743–51.

28. Lim BL, Kelly AM. A meta-analysis on the utility of peripheral venous blood gas analyses in exacerbations of chronic obstructive pulmonary disease in the emergency department. Eur J Emerg Med 2010;17(5):246–8.

29. Kelly AM. Agreement between arterial and venous blood gases in emergency medical care: a systematic review Hong Kong. J Emerg Med 2013;20:166–71.

30. Kelly AM, Kerr D, Middleton P. Validation of venous pCO2 to screen for arterial hypercarbia in patients with chronic obstructive airways disease. J Emerg Med 2005;28:377–9.

31. Kelly AM, Kyle E, McAlpine R. Venous pCO2 and pH can be used to screen for significant hypercarbia in emergency patients with acute respiratory disease. J Emerg Med 2002;22:15–9.

32. Sur E. COPD: is it all in the vein? Thorax 2013;68(Suppl 3):P182.

33. McCanny P, Bennett K, Staunton P, et al. Venous vs. arterial blood gases in the assessment of patients presenting with an exacerbation of chronic obstructive pulmonary disease. Am J Emerg Med 2012;30:896–900.

34. Ibrahim I, Ooi SBS, Huak CY, et al. Point-of-care bedside gas analyzer: limited use of venous pCO2 in emergency patients. J Emerg Med 2011;41:117–23.

35. Domaradzki L, Gosala S, Iskandarani K, et al. Is venous blood gas performed in the Emergency Department predictive of outcome during acute on chronic hypercarbic respiratory failure? Clin Respir J 2018;12(5):1849–57.

36. Dogan NO, S ener A, Gunaydin GP, et al. The accuracy of mainstream end-tidal carbon dioxide levels to predict the severity of chronic obstructive pulmonary disease exacerbations presented to the ED. Am J Emerg Med 2014;32(5): 408–11.

37. Cinar O, Acar YA, Arziman I, et al. Can mainstream end-tidal carbon dioxide measurement accurately predict the arterial carbon dioxide level of patients with acute dyspnea in ED. Am J Emerg Med 2012;30:358–61.

38. Long B, Koyfman A, Vivirito MA. Capnography in the Emergency Department: A Review of Uses, Waveforms, and Limitations. J Emerg Med 2017;53(6):829–42.

39. Nik Hisamuddin NA, Rashidi A, Chew KS, et al. Correlations between capnographic waveforms and peak flow meter measurement in emergency department management of asthma. Int J Emerg Med 2009;2(2):83–9.

40. You B, Peslin R, Duvivier C, et al. Expiratory capnography in asthma: evaluation of various shape indices. Eur Respir J 1994;7(2):318–23.

41. Yaron M, Padyk P, Hutsinpiller M, et al. Utility of the expiratory capnogram in the assessment of bronchospasm. Ann Emerg Med 1996;28:403–7.

42. Howe TA, Jaalam K, Ahmad R, et al. The use of end-tidal capnography to monitor non-intubated patients presenting with acute exacerbation of asthma in the emergency department. J Emerg Med 2011;41:581–9.

43. Murray CJ, Atkinson C, Bhalla K, et al. The State of US health, 1990-2010: burden of diseases, injuries, and risk factors. JAMA 2013;310:591–608.

44. Curkendall SM, DeLuise C, Jones JK, et al. Cardiovascular disease in patients with chronic obstructive pulmonary disease, Saskatchewan Canada cardiovascular disease in COPD patients. Ann Epidemiol 2006;16:63–70.

45. Schneider C, Bothner U, Jick SS, et al. Chronic obstructive pulmonary disease and the risk of cardiovascular diseases. Eur J Epidemiol 2010;25:253–60.

46. Khalid N, Chhabra L, Spodick DH. Electrocardiographic screening of emphysema: lead aVL or Leads III and I? Acta Inform Med 2013;21(3):223.

47. Rodman DM, Lowenstein SR, Rodman T. The electrocardiogram in chronic obstructive pulmonary disease. J Emerg Med 1990;8:607–15.

48. Shah NS, Koller SM, Janower ML, et al. Diaphragm levels as determinants of P axis in restrictive vs obstructive pulmonary disease. Chest 1995;107(3):697–700.

49. Thomas AJ, Apiyasawat S, Spodick DH. Electrocardiographic detection of emphysema. Am J Cardiol 2011;107:1090–2.

50. Friedman PJ. Imaging studies in emphysema. Proc Am Thorac Soc 2008;5:494–500.

51. Tsai T, Gallagher E, Lombardi G, et al. Guidelines for the selective ordering of admission chest radiography in adult obstructive airway disease. Ann Emerg Med 1993;22:1854–8.

52. Washko GR. Diagnostic imaging in COPD. Semin Respir Crit Care Med 2010;31:276–85.

53. Wallace GM, Winter JH, Winter JE, et al. Chest x-rays in COPD screening: are they worthwhile? Respir Med 2009;103:1862–5.

54. Staub LJ, Mazzali Biscaro RR, Kaszubowski E, et al. Lung ultrasound for the emergency diagnosis of pneumonia, acute heart failure, and exacerbations of chronic obstructive pulmonary disease/asthma in adults: a systematic review and meta-analysis. J Emerg Med 2019;56:53–69.

55. Doerschug KC, Schmidt GA. Intensive care ultrasound: III. Lung and pleural ultrasound for the intensivist. Ann Am Thorac Soc 2013;10:708–12.

56. Lichtenstein D, van Hooland S, Elbers P, et al. Ten good reasons to practice ultrasound in critical care. Anaesthesiol Intensive Ther 2014;46(5):323–35.

57. Gallard E, Redonnet JP, Bourcier JE, et al. Diagnostic performance of cardiopulmonary ultrasound performed by the emergency physician in the management of acute dyspnea. Am J Emerg Med 2015;33(3):352–8.

58. Silva S, Biendel C, Ruiz J, et al. Usefulness of cardiothoracic chest ultrasound in the management of acute respiratory failure in critical care practice. Chest 2013; 144(3):859–65.

59. Sellers WFS. Inhaled and intravenous treatment in acute severe and life threatening asthma. Br J Anaesth 2013;110(2):183–90.

60. Chien JW, Ciufo R, Novak R, et al. Uncontrolled oxygen administration and respiratory failure in acute asthma. Chest 2000;117:728–33.

61. Rodrigo GJ, Rodriquez Verde M, Peregalli V, et al. Effects of short-term 28% and 100% oxygen on PaCO2 and peak expiratory flow rate in acute asthma: a randomized trial. Chest 2003;124:1312–7.

62. Perrin K, Wijesinghe M, Healy B, et al. Randomised controlled trial of high concentration versus titrated oxygen therapy in severe exacerbations of asthma. Thorax 2011;66:937–41.

63. Sassoon CSH, Hassell KT, Mahutte CK. Hypoxic induced hypercapnia in stable chronic obstructive pulmonary disease. Am Rev Respir Dis 1987;135:907–11.

64. Susanto C, Thomas PS. Assessing the use of initial oxygen therapy in chronic obstructive pulmonary disease patients: a retrospective audit of pre-hospital and hospital emergency management. Intern Med J 2015;45(5):510–6.

65. Austin M, Wills E, Blizzard L, et al. Effect of high flow oxygen on mortality on chronic obstructive pulmonary disease patients in prehospital setting: randomized controlled trial. BMJ 2010;341:c546.

66. Beasley R, Aldington S, Robinson G. Is it time to change the approach to oxygen therapy in the breathless patient? Thorax 2007;62:840–1.

67. Cates CJ, Crilly JA, Rowe BH. Holding chambers (spacers) versus nebulisers for beta-agonist treatment of acute asthma. Cochrane Database Syst Rev 2006;(2):CD000052.

68. Turner MO, Gafni A, Swan D, et al. A review and economic evaluation of bronchodilator delivery methods in hospitalized patients. Arch Intern Med 1996;156: 2113–8.

69. Ameredes BT, Calhoun WJ. Albuterol enantiomers: pre-clinical and clinical value? Front Biosci (Elite Ed 2010;2:1081–92.

70. Andrews T, McGintee E, Mittal MK, et al. High-dose continuous nebulized levalbuterol for pediatric status asthmaticus: a randomized trial. J Pediatr 2009;155: 205–10.

71. Wilkinson M, Bulloch B, Garcia-Filion P, et al. Efficacy of racemic albuterol versus levalbuterol used as a continuous nebulization for the treatment of acute asthma exacerbations: a randomized, double-blind, clinical trial. J Asthma 2011;48(2):188–93.

72. Jat KR, Khairwa A. Levalbuterol versus albuterol for acute asthma: A systematic review and meta-analysis. Pulm Pharmacol Ther 2013;26(2):239–48.

73. Rowe BH. Continuous versus intermittent beta-agonists for acute asthma. Cochrane Database Syst Rev 2011;4:CD001115.

74. Castle W, Fuller R, Hall J, et al. Serevent nationwide surveillance study: comparison of salmeterol with salbutamol in asthmatic patients who require regular bronchodilator treatment. BMJ 1993;306:1034–7.

75. Nelson HS, Weiss ST, Bleecker ER, et al. The salmeterol multicenter asthma research trial: a comparison of usual pharmacotherapy for asthma or usual pharmacotherapy plus salmeterol. Chest 2006;129:15–26.

76. Mann M, Chowdhury B, Sullivan E, et al. Serious asthma exacerbations in asthmatics treated with high-dose formoterol. Chest 2003;124:70–4.

77. Horita N, Goto A, Shibata Y, et al. Long-acting muscarinic antagonist (LAMA) plus long-acting beta-agonist (LABA) versus LABA plus inhaled corticosteroid (ICS) for stable chronic obstructive pulmonary disease (COPD). Cochrane Database Syst Rev 2017;2:CD012066.
78. Rogliani P, Calzetta L, Braido F, et al. LABA/LAMA fixed-dose combinations in patients with COPD: a systematic review. Int J Chron Obstruct Pulmon Dis 2018;13:3115–30.
79. Criner GL, Bourbeau J, Diekemper RL, et al. Prevention of Acute Exacerbations of COPD: American College of Chest Physicians and Canadian Thoracic Society Guideline. Chest 2015;147(4):894–942.
80. Maia IS, Pincelli MP, Leite VF, et al. Long acting muscarinic antagonists vs. long-acting beta 2 agonists in COPD exacerbations: a systematic review and meta-analysis. J Bras Pneumol 2017;43:302–12.
81. Price D, Yawn B, Brusselle G, et al. Risk-to-benefit ratio of inhaled corticosteroids in patients with COPD. Prim Care Respir J 2013;22:92–100.
82. Adoun M, Frat JP, Doré P, et al. Comparison of nebulized epinephrine and terbutaline in patients with acute severe asthma: a controlled trial. J Crit Care 2004;19(2):99–102.
83. Coupe MO, Guly U, Brown E, et al. Nebulised adrenaline in acute severe asthma: comparison with salbutamol. Eur J Respir Dis 1987;71(4):227–32.
84. Plint AC, Osmond MH, Klassen TP. The efficacy of nebulized racemic epinephrine in children with acute asthma: a randomized, double-blind trial. Acad Emerg Med 2000;7(10):1097–103.
85. Abroug F, Nouira S, Bchir A, et al. A controlled trial of nebulized salbutamol and adrenaline in acute severe asthma. Intensive Care Med 1995;21(1):18–23.
86. Zeggwagh AA, Abouqal R, Madani N, et al. [Comparative efficiency of nebulized adrenaline and salbutamol in severe acute asthma. A randomized, controlled prospective study]. Ann Fr Anesth Reanim 2002;21(9):703–9.
87. Rennard SI. Treatment of stable chronic obstructive pulmonary disease. Lancet 2004;364(9436):791–802.
88. Rodrigo GJ, Castro-Rodriguez JA. Anticholinergics in the treatment of children and adults with acute asthma: a systematic review with meta-analysis. Thorax 2005;60:740–6.
89. Plotnick LH, Ducharme FM. Acute asthma in children and adolescents: should inhaled anticholinergics be added to beta(2)-agonists? Am J Respir Med 2003;2:109–15.
90. Zorc JJ, Pusic MV, Ogborn CJ, et al. Ipratropium bromide added to asthma treatment in the pediatric emergency department. Pediatrics 1999;103(4 Pt 1): 748–52.
91. Stoodley RG, Aaron SD, Dales RE. The role of ipratropium bromide in the emergency management of acute asthma exacerbation: a metaanalysis of randomized clinical trials. Ann Emerg Med 1999;34:8–18.
92. Vezina K, Chauhan BF, Ducharme FM. Inhaled anticholinergics and short-acting beta(2)-agonists versus short-acting beta2-agonists alone for children with acute asthma in hospital. Cochrane Database Syst Rev 2014;7:CD010283.
93. Griffiths B, Ducharme FM. Combined inhaled anticholinergics and short-acting beta2-agonists for initial treatment of acute asthma in children. Cochrane Database Syst Rev 2013;(8):CD000060.
94. Kerstjens HA, Engel M, Dahl R, et al. Tiotropium in asthma poorly controlled with standard combination therapy. N Engl J Med 2012;367:1198–207.

95. VA/DoD Clinical Practice Guidelines. Management of Chronic Obstructive Pulmonary Disease (COPD). 2021. Available at: https://www.healthquality.va.gov/guidelines/cd/copd/. Accessed September 1, 2021.

96. Rowe BH, Spooner CH, Ducharme FM, et al. Corticosteroids for preventing relapse following acute exacerbations of asthma. Cochrane Database Syst Rev 2007;(3):CD000195.

97. Edmonds ML, Milan SJ, Camargo CA Jr, et al. Early use of inhaled corticosteroids in the emergency department treatment of acute asthma. Cochrane Database Syst Rev 2012;12:CD002308.

98. Walters JA, Tan DJ, White CJ, et al. Systemic corticosteroids for acute exacerbations of chronic obstructive pulmonary disease. Cochrane Database Syst Rev 2014;9:CD001288.

99. Mendes ES, Cadet L, Arana J, et al. Acute effect of an inhaled glucocorticosteroid on albuterol-induced bronchodilation in patients with moderately severe asthma. Chest 2015;147(4):1037–42.

100. Alia I, de la Cal MA, Esteban A, et al. Efficacy of corticosteroid therapy in patients with an acute exacerbation of chronic obstructive pulmonary disease receiving ventilatory support. Arch Intern Med 2011;171:1939–46.

101. Schacke H, Docke WD, Asadullah K. Mechanisms involved in the side effects of glucocorticoids. Pharmacol Ther 2002;96:23–43.

102. Cheng T, Gong Y, Guo Y, et al. Systemic corticosteroid for COPD exacerbations, whether the higher dose is better? A meta-analysis of randomized controlled trials. Clin Respir J 2013;7:305–18.

103. Schacke H, Schottelius A, Docke WD, et al. Dissociation of transactivation from transrepression by a selective glucocorticoid receptor agonist leads to separation of therapeutic effects from side effects. Proc Natlacadsciusa 2004;101:227–32.

104. Kiser TH, Allen RR, Valuck RJ, et al. Outcomes associated with corticosteroid dosage in critically ill patients with acute exacerbations of chronic obstructive pulmonary disease. Am J Respir Crit Care Med 2014;189:1052–64.

105. Leuppi JD, Schuetz P, Bingisser R, et al. Short-term vs conventional glucocorticoid therapy in acute exacerbations of chronic obstructive pulmonary disease: the REDUCE randomized clinical trial. JAMA 2013;309:2223–31.

106. Kew KM, Kirtchuk L, Michell CI. Intravenous magnesium sulfate for treating adults with acute asthma in the emergency department. Cochrane Database Syst Rev 2014;(5):CD010909.

107. Alter HJ, Koepsell TD, Hilty WM. Intravenous magnesium as an adjuvant in acute bronchospasm: a meta-analysis. Ann Emerg Med 2000;36:191–7.

108. Rowe BH, Bretzlaff JA, Bourdon C, et al. Intravenous magnesium sulfate treatment for acute asthma in the emergency department: a systematic review of the literature. Ann Emerg Med 2000;36:181–90.

109. Hirashima J, Yamana H, Matsui H, et al. Effect of intravenous magnesium sulfate on mortality in patients with severe acute asthma. Respirology 2016;21(4):668–73.

110. Knightly R, Milan SJ, Hughes R, et al. Inhaled magnesium sulfate in the treatment of acute asthma. Cochrane Database Syst Rev 2017;11:Cd003898.

111. Su Z, Li R, Gai Z. Intravenous and Nebulized Magnesium Sulfate for Treating Acute Asthma in Children: A Systematic Review and Meta-Analysis. Pediatr Emerg Care 2018;34(6):390–5.

112. Goyal S, Agrawal A. Ketamine in status asthmaticus: a review. Indian J Crit Care Med 2013;17(3):154–61.

113. Sato T, Hirota K, Matsuki A, et al. The role of the N-Methyl-D-Aspartic acid receptor in the relaxant effect of ketamine on tracheal smooth muscle. Anesth Analg 1998;87:1383–8.
114. Zhu MM, Qian YN, Zhu W, et al. Protective effects of ketamine on allergenin-duced airway inflammatory injure and high airway reactivity in asthma: experiment with rats. Zhonghua Yi Xue Za Zhi 2007;87:1308–13.
115. Shlamovitz GZ, Hawthorne T. Intravenous ketamine in a dissociating dose as a temporizing measure to avoid mechanical ventilation in adult patient with severe asthma exacerbation. J Emerg Med 2011;41(5):492–4.
116. Youssef-Ahmed MZ, Silver P, Nimkoff L, et al. Continuous infusion of ketamine in mechanically ventilated children with refractory bronchospasm. Intensive Care Med 1996;22(9):972–6.
117. Smith D, Riel J, Tilles I, et al. Intravenous epinephrine in life-threatening asthma. Ann Emerg Med 2003;41(5):706–11.
118. Travers AH, Milan SJ, Jones AP, et al. Addition of intravenous beta(2)-agonists to inhaled beta(2)-agonists for acute asthma. Cochrane Database Syst Rev 2012; 12:CD010179.
119. Cydulka R, Davison R, Grammer L, et al. The use of epinephrine in the treatment of older adult asthmatics. Ann Emerg Med 1988;17(4):322–6.
120. Lee DL, Lee H, Chang HW, et al. Heliox improves hemodynamics in mechanically ventilated patients with chronic obstructive pulmonary disease with systolic pressure variations. Crit Care Med 2005;33(5):968–73.
121. El-Khatib MF, Jamaleddine G. Effect of heliox- and air-driven nebulized broncho-dilator therapy on lung function in patients with asthma. Lung 2014;192:377–83.
122. Rodrigo GJ, Rodriguez-Castro JA. Heliox-driven b2-agonists nebulization for children and adults with acute asthma: a systematic review with meta-analysis. Ann Allergy Asthma Immunol 2014;112:29–34.
123. Ram FS, Rodriguez-Roisin R, Granados-Navarrete A, et al. Antibiotics for exacerbations of chronic obstructive pulmonary disease. Cochrane Database Syst Rev 2006;19(2):CD004403.
124. Domenech A, Puig C, Marti S, et al. Infectious etiology of acute exacerbations in severe COPD patients. J Infect 2013;67:516–23.
125. Decramer M, Janssens W, Miravitlles M. Chronic obstructive pulmonary disease. Lancet 2012;379:1341–51.
126. Sethi S, Murphy TF. Infection in the pathogenesis and course of chronic obstructive pulmonary disease. N Engl J Med 2008;359:2355–65.
127. White AJ, Gompertz S, Bayley DL, et al. Resolution of bronchial inflammation is related to bacterial eradication following treatment of exacerbations of chronic bronchitis. Thorax 2003;58:680–5.
128. Siddiqi A, Sethi S. Optimizing antibiotic selection in treating COPD exacerbations. Int J Chron Obstruct Pulmon Dis 2008;3:31.
129. Mallia P, Johnston SL. Influenza infection and COPD. Int J Chron Obstruct Pulmon Dis 2007;2:55–64.
130. Buda AJ, Pinsky MR, Ingels NB Jr, et al. Effect of intrathoracic pressure on left ventricular performance. N Engl J Med 1979;301:453–9.
131. Stather DR, Stewart TE. Clinical review: Mechanical ventilation in severe asthma. Crit Care 2005;9(6):581–7.
132. Broux R, Foidart G, Mendes P, et al. Use of PEEP in management of life-threatening status asthmaticus: a method for the recovery of appropriate ventilation perfusion ratio. Appl Cardiopulm Pathophysiol 1991;4:79–83.

133. Lim WJ, Mohammed Akram R, Carson KV, et al. Noninvasive positive & pressure ventilation for treatment of respiratory failure due to severe acute exacerbations of asthma. Cochrane Database Syst Rev 2012;12:CD004360.

134. Ameen A, Zedan M, El Shamly M. Comparison between continuous positive airway pressure and bilevel positive pressure ventilation in treatment of acute exacerbation of chronic obstructive pulmonary disease. Egypt J Chest Dis Tuberc 2012;61:95–101.

135. Wedzicha JAEC-C, Miravitlles M, Hurst JR, et al. Management of COPD exacerbations: a European Respiratory Society/American Thoracic Society guideline. Eur Respir J 2017;49:1600791.

136. Bond KR, Horsley CA, Williams AB. Non-invasive ventilation use in status asthmaticus: 16 years of experience in a tertiary intensive care. Emerg Med Australas 2018;30(2):187–92.

137. Althoff MD, Holguin F, Yang F, et al. Noninvasive Ventilation Use in Critically Ill Patients with Acute Asthma Exacerbations. Am J Respir Crit Care Med 2020; 202(11):1520–30, d.

138. Weingart SD. Managing Initial Mechanical Ventilation in the Emergency Department. Ann Emerg Med 2016;68(5):614–7.

139. Lodeserto FJ, Lettich TM, Rezaie SR. High-flow Nasal Cannula: Mechanisms of Action and Adult and Pediatric Indications. Cureus 2018;10(11):e3639.

140. Long B, Liang SY, Lentz S. High flow nasal cannula for adult acute hypoxemic respiratory failure in the ED setting: A narrative review. Am J Emerg Med 2021;49:352–9.

141. Nishimura M. High-flow nasal cannula oxygen therapy in adults. J Intensive Care 2015;3:15.

142. Crisafulli E, Barbeta E, Ielpo A, et al. Management of severe acute exacerbations of COPD: an updated narrative review. Multidiscip Respir Med 2018;13:36.

143. Pisani L, Astuto M, Prediletto I, et al. High flow through nasal cannula in exacerbated COPD patients: a systematic review. Pulmonology 2019;25(6):348–54.

144. Bruni A, Garofalo E, Cammarota G, et al. High Flow Through Nasal Cannula in Stable and Exacerbated Chronic Obstructive Pulmonary Disease Patients. Rev Recent Clin Trials 2019;14(4):247–60.

145. Murase K, Tomii K, Chin K, et al. The use of non-invasive ventilation for life threatening asthma attacks: changes in the need for intubation. Respirology 2010;15: 714–20.

146. Brenner B, Corbridge T, Kazzi A. Intubation and mechanical ventilation of the patient in respiratory failure. J Emerg Med 2009;37(2S):S23–34.

147. Braman SS, Kaemmerlen JT. Intensive care of status asthmaticus. A 10-year experience. JAMA 1990;264:366–8.

148. Weingart SD, Levitan RM. Preoxygenation and prevention of desaturation during emergency airway management. Ann Emerg Med 2012;59(3):165–75.e1.

149. Weingart SD. Preoxygenation, reoxygenation, and delayed sequence intubation in the emergency department. J Emerg Med 2011;40(6):661–7.

150. Brown RH, Wagner EM. Mechanisms of bronchoprotection by anesthetic induction agents: propofol versus ketamine. Anesthesiology 1999;90:822–8.

151. Perry JJ, Lee JS, Sillberg VA, et al. Rocuronium versus succinylcholine for rapid sequence induction intubation. Cochrane Database Syst Rev 2008;(2): CD002788.

152. Lougheed MD, Fisher T, O'Donnell DE. Dynamic hyperinflation during bronchoconstriction in asthma: implications for symptom perception. Chest 2006;130: 1072–81.

53. Schauer SG, Cuenca PJ, Johnson JJ, et al. Management of acute asthma in the emergency department. Emerg Med Pract 2013;15(6):1–28.
54. Adnet F, Racine SX, Lapostolle F, et al. Full reversal of hypercapnic coma by noninvasive positive pressure ventilation. Am J Emerg Med 2001;19:244–6.
55. Yeo HJ, Kim D, Jeon D, et al. Extracorporeal membrane oxygenation for life-threatening asthma refractory to mechanical ventilation: analysis of the Extracorporeal Life Support Organization registry. Crit Care 2017;21(1):297.

Diagnosis and Management of Pulmonary Embolism

Terren Trott, MD[a,b,]*, Jason Bowman, MD[b]

KEYWORDS

- Pulmonary embolism • Cardiac arrest • Thrombolysis

KEY POINTS

- Presenting symptoms of pulmonary emboli can be nonspecific, and maintaining a high level of suspicion is appropriate for the evaluation of emergency department patients.
- Using clinical decision tools such as the Wells criteria and the PERC rule can safely rule out pulmonary embolism in a substantial portion of patients.
- Newer data have shown the safety of using an age-adjusted d-dimer approach and the YEARS criteria.
- Bedside echocardiography has value in prognosticating confirmed pulmonary emboli but is not necessarily as useful for making a diagnosis.
- Management of submassive pulmonary emboli remains controversial and may include catheter-directed thrombolysis, systemic thrombolysis, or anticoagulation alone.

INTRODUCTION

Acute pulmonary embolism (PE) is a relatively common form of venous thromboembolism that can lead to significant morbidity and mortality, with additional legal liability for emergency providers if it is not quickly diagnosed and treated **Figs. 1–5**. PEs can occur in both the young and old, are not limited to their common presentations, and can frequently present with unusual chief complaints. Pairing this with desire to limit contrast injury, radiation, and complications of anticoagulation can make the diagnosis and treatment of PEs challenging. In this article, we discuss the epidemiology, classifications, approach, and management of this challenging disease.

Authors have nothing to disclose.
a Department of Emergency Medicine, University of Kentucky, 800 Rose Street, Lexington, KY 40503, USA; b Department of Pulmonary, Critical Care and Sleep Medicine, University of Kentucky, 800 Rose Street, Lexington, KY 40503, USA
* Corresponding author. Department of Emergency Medicine, University of Kentucky, 800 Rose Street, Lexington, KY 40503.
E-mail address: terren.trott@gmail.com

Emerg Med Clin N Am 40 (2022) 565–581
https://doi.org/10.1016/j.emc.2022.05.008
0733-8627/22/Published by Elsevier Inc.

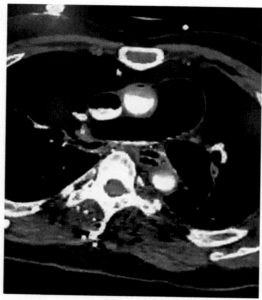

Fig. 1. A CT image showing an air emboli.

EPIDEMIOLOGY/PREVALENCE/INCIDENCE

With 500,000 to 600,000 diagnoses a year and an estimated 200,000 to 300,000 deaths a year, PE imparts a substantial global burden of disease. The world incidence is approximately 0.75 to 2.69 per 1000 people, with an estimated 4.2 per 1000 people in the United States.[1] Incidence is notably higher in the elderly population with up to three times the diagnoses in patients over 70 year old or 13.8 per 1000 people in patients over 65.[2] Venothromboembolism does not discriminate across high-, middle-, and low-income countries[3] and has a significant impact on morbidity with the reduction in healthy-life years lost and reduction in long-term survival.[4] It is also estimated

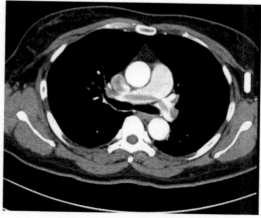

Fig. 2. A CT scan showing a saddle pulmonary embolism.

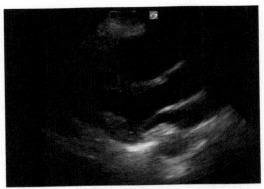

Fig. 3. A parasternal long-axis view with dilation of the right ventricle. This can grossly be assessed by seeing the diameter is greater than the aorta or the left atrium.

that 5% to 10% of in-hospital deaths are secondary to PE, again in most of the patients over 60 year old.[5] This is likely secondary to the increased risk of venous thromboembolic (VTE) in hospitalized patients.[4]

CLASSIFICATION

There are multiple approaches to the classification of PE and their interchangeable usage can lead to some confusion. Pulmonary embolic events can be classified by acuity, origin, anatomic location, and severity.

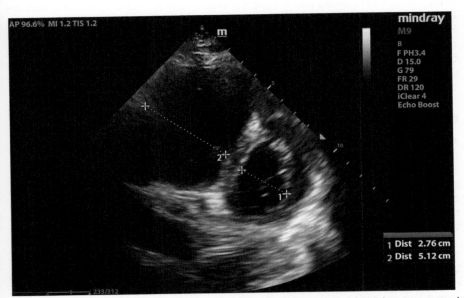

Fig. 4. A parasternal short axis. Here, the intraventricular chambers have been measured and showed a gross enlargement of the right ventricle. A "D-sign" can also be see with compression of the septum into the left ventricle.

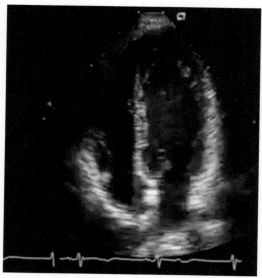

Fig. 5. A normal apical four-chamber view without ventricular dilation.

CLASSIFICATION BASED ON ACUITY

The most broad classification category can be found in acuity. The acute PE can frequently be fatal, symptomatic, or even silent. The majority of this review focuses on acute PE, an imperative diagnosis for the emergency practitioner. Acute PEs are also frequently classified by their origin and/or severity. Subacute PE refers to the patient who presents 2 to 12 weeks after the onset of initial symptoms. Although not as symptomatic as the acute PE, still carries a high mortality and high risk of conversion to the chronic PE and associated chronic thromboembolic pulmonary hypertension (CTEPH). The chronic form of PE is classified as pulmonary hypertension (WHO group 4) for at least 6 months following an acute PE. Frequently, however, an acute embolic event goes undiagnosed leading to a chronic clot burden in the pulmonary vasculature which can be difficult, if not impossible, to accurately diagnose in the emergency department.

CLASSIFICATION BASED ON ORIGIN

Acute PEs can be classified as in situ or embolic. Embolic can further be classified as thrombotic or non-thrombotic in nature with thromboembolic being by far the most common. The idea of in situ pulmonary thrombosis as a response to local lung injury is relatively new.[6] Clinically, it would warrant a unique treatment plan as it could be considered a provoked thrombus and therefore could be treated with a shorter duration pending elimination of the triggering insult. In situ pulmonary thrombosis is postulated to be the primary cause of pulmonary emboli related to COVID-19 pneumonia.[7]

VTE events are the primary cause of PEs and typically originate as a deep venous thrombosis with subsequent migration into the pulmonary vasculature. The risk for VTE is a combination of the individual's risk factors, such as inborn coagulopathies combined with any triggering conditions, such as the presence of malignancy, shock, recent immobilization, injury, and other risk factors like hormone replacement or tobacco use. Non-thrombotic emboli are less common and are associated with conditions such as amniotic embolism with peripartum state, fat emboli with long bone fracture, septic emboli with endocarditic valvular vegetations, tumor emboli with malignancy, foreign body emboli with instrumentation, and air emboli with central or even peripheral vascular access complications.

CLASSIFICATION BASED ON ANATOMIC LOCATION

Radiographic reports, understandably, often describe the anatomic location of the pulmonary embolus as saddle, lobar, segmental, or subsegmental and then list any associated findings such as evidence of right heart strain. Clot in transit is an uncommon location-based finding but is associated with a high mortality of 27%.[8]

Saddle embolus is typically used to refer to an emboli that is resting on the bifurcation of the right and left pulmonary artery. Saddle emboli are frequently associated with hemodynamic instability and carry an independent mortality of approximately 5%. Occasionally, however, the term saddle emboli may be used to identify an embolus resting on the bifurcation of a lesser artery in the pulmonary tree, if this use of the term saddle emboli is found in the radiology report, care must be taken to ensure this is well communicated to avoid unnecessary interventions from taking place.

A lobar embolus is located in one of the six lobar branches of the pulmonary artery. These branches arise from the main pulmonary arteries and typically consist of the upper, middle, and lower branches of the right pulmonary artery, or the upper, lingular, and lower branches of the left pulmonary artery. These branches frequently accompany their associated bronchi.

The lobar pulmonary arteries continue to branch into the segmental and then subsegmental pulmonary arteries; typically, 17 branches are present but significant variability exists between patients, and identification of the associated airways is usually required to identify the affected branch. To identify a subsegmental PE (SSPE), the radiologist must identify the presence of a subsegmental vessel and note a filling defect within it. On its own an SSPE is relatively innocuous; however, widespread SSPE can be quite symptomatic. This leads clinicians to the use of a severity-based classification system.

CLASSIFICATION BASED ON SEVERITY

Probably the most useful classification for clinicians, and the one recommended by most clinical treatment guidelines, is the severity-based classification. There are three categories of severity, massive/high-risk, submassive/intermediate-risk, and small/low-risk pulmonary emboli.

Massive or high-risk pulmonary emboli are characterized by hemodynamic instability, that is, a systolic blood pressure less than 90 mm Hg requiring vasopressor support. As multiple small emboli in a relatively baseline debilitated individual could be called a "massive PE," the risk-based naming convention has come about because of the inherent confusion with the use of the word massive to mean very symptomatic, rather than refer to the actual size of the embolus.

In the hemodynamically stable subset, submassive or intermediate-risk and small or low-risk pulmonary emboli are distinguished by the presence or absence of right ventricular strain on computed tomography (CT) or echocardiography or the presence or absence of elevated cardiac troponins.

CLASSIFICATION BASED ON CAUSE

One additional descriptor to be mindful of when discussing long-term therapy choices is the presence of underlying long-term coagulopathy versus short-term coagulopathy. Frequently described as whether the thrombotic event was provoked or unprovoked. For example, a PE that occurs after an overseas international flight, or after surgery or hospitalization would be considered provoked. Whereas a PE that occurs with no defining cause or attributed to the presence of a chronic disease state such as chronic obstructive pulmonary disease (COPD) or heart disease would be considered unprovoked.

CLINICAL PRESENTATION OF PULMONARY EMBOLISM

Diagnosis of PE can be challenging because of the nonspecific nature of many clinical and even laboratory findings. The complexity of diagnosis is secondary to the pathophysiology, multiple risk factors, organ systems involved as well as the breadth of severity of the clinical presentation of PE. Clinical findings range from sudden cardiac death to signs and symptoms of paradoxic emboli to an entirely asymptomatic presentation.[6] Historical data such as prior VTE, recent surgery or immobilization, cancer, obesity, and pregnancy confer increased risk; however, even approximately 30% of patients will present with no known risk factors.[9]

Cardiac Arrest

Registry data suggest that 3% of patients admitted alive after sudden cardiac death suffered arrest from a massive PE. When compared with non-PE-related death, those diagnosed with PE were more likely to present without a shockable rhythm (6% vs 50%, OR 12.4), more likely to be women (71% vs 46%), and more likely to have a prior diagnosis of venothromboembolism (23% vs 3%). In this study, the absence of a non-shockable rhythm and prior VTE had an NPV of 98% for ruling out the diagnosis of massive PE.[10,11]

Noncardiac Arrest

Slightly less dramatic presentations may include the signs and symptoms of shock and right ventricular failure. Right ventricular function plays a central role in management and classification but also in clinical presentation. Significant dyspnea, hypotension, tachycardia, and hypoxia may be present when the right ventricle is impaired. Shock is present in 5% to 10% of these patients and an elevated shock index is often present.[9,12] An elevated shock index (>1.0) has been shown to correlate moderately well with in-patient mortality (OR 5.8), myocardial necrosis (OR 5.0), and very well with right ventricular dysfunction (OR 53.5).[13]

Syncope comprises 6% to 35% of initial chief complaints of PE but is a rather nonspecific and common emergency department presentation. Syncope is also more common in massive and submassive PE. Several mechanisms have been proposed to explain syncope including a sudden reduction in cardiac output leading to decreased cerebral perfusion and arrhythmias. A vasovagal response has also been proposed in response to sudden thrombosis causing a stretch on ventricular mechanoreceptors leading to an increase in the efferent vagal response, bradycardia, and decrease in sympathetic tone and subsequent syncope.[14]

Chest pain is a common symptom in PE; however, quality of pain may vary based on the underlying pathology. Pleuritic pain may be present with pulmonary infarction or pleural irritation, whereas anginal symptoms or epigastric pain may result from RV dysfunction or myocardial infarction. Chest pain may be associated with a cough or dyspnea. Distribution of symptoms varies from study to study and severity of disease; however, the most recent registry data found a distribution of dyspnea (50%), chest pain (54%), pleuritic pain (39%), cough (23%), respiratory distress (16%), fever (10%), and hemoptysis (8%).[1]

APPROACH TO DIAGNOSIS

The electrocardiogram is ubiquitously performed in patients presenting with chest pain and shortness of breath; however, it also suffers from poor sensitivity and specificity in aiding the diagnosis of PE. In fact, approximately 25% of electrocardiograms (ECGs) will be normal at times of presentation.[15] The most common findings are sinus tachycardia and precordial lead t-wave inversions.[15,16] Findings may also include right bundle branch block, right axis deviation, atrial dysrhythmias, and right ventricular strain pattern. The classic findings of prominent S-wave in lead I, with Q-waves and inverted T-waves in lead III, are a rare finding (3%–25% sensitive) with the highest reported specificity at 51%[15,17] in acute PE. The test characteristics of this finding may be increased with significant RV strain or in syncope associated presentations.[17]

Given the limited utility of clinical and ECG findings in cinching the diagnosis of PE, clinical decision-making tools in conjunction with d-dimer laboratory testing is often used. The PERC criteria and WELLS criteria are well validated and widely used, whereas more recent studies have aimed at reducing CT utilization with novel d-dimer cutoff values. The PERC criteria have been validated to rule out PE to less than 2% likelihood in low suspicion patients, defined as pretest probability less than 15%.[18,19] Alternatively to physician gestalt, the WELLS criteria can also aid in identifying low-risk patients and are often used in conjunction with the PERC criteria.[20,21] In patients with a negative d-dimer and low-risk WELLS score or WELLS low-risk and PERC negative, PE can be safely excluded.

Newer algorithms have investigated the utility of an age-adjusted d-dimer limit in low- and moderate-risk patients. The original age-adjusted d-dimer method was studied in 2013 and used a cutoff of limit of age x 10 ng/mL in patients over 50 year old. This meta-analysis study of over 12,000 patients showed increased specificity at each decade stratum when compared conventional cutoff values allowing for more selective CT imaging.[22] A prospective, multicenter validation study of 3346 patients confirmed the age-adjusted cutoff values with only one missed case of PE.[23] A retrospective study of an age-adjusted d-dimer showed a small reduction in sensitivity but also showed a substantial reduction in unnecessary CT imaging.[23,24]

The YEARS criteria are also a novel and simplified approach to diagnosis and exclusion of PE. The landmark multicenter, prospective study examined 3465 patients using three clinical criteria: signs of DVT, hemoptysis, or PE as most likely diagnosis, in conjunction with a d-dimer. In the absence of any of these three findings, a d-dimer cutoff of 1000 ng/mL safely ruled out PE.[25] A prospective observational study showed very promising test characteristics with a near 100% NPV.[26] Although both the age-adjusted d-dimer cutoff and YEARS criteria are promising to increase efficiency in the emergency department, both are relatively recent advances in the diagnosis of PE.

BEDSIDE TRANSTHORACIC ECHOCARDIOGRAPHY

The availability and immediacy of bedside transthoracic echocardiography can be useful in the immediate resuscitative phase of patients in profound shock to identify acute cor pulmonale, which can be attributed to a massive PE in the proper clinical context. The four cardiac views, the parasternal long axis, parasternal short axis, the apical four chamber, and the subxiphoid view are typically used when assessing right ventricular function. Assessment is typically centered around volume changes, decreased systolic function, or signs of acute pressure change. Each view can offer insight into these changes.

In the parasternal long-axis view, RV dilation may be observed. Using a general rule of thumb that the left atrium, aortic outflow tract, and the RV outflow track can be a quick visual method of identifying a dilated RV. However, once dilation is suspected, it should be confirmed in other views as well.

The parasternal short axis is useful for assessing both dilation of the RV and signs of increased pressure. In the short axis, at the level of the papillaries or mitral valve, the RV diameter should be 0.6:1 with respect to the LV diameter. Ratios greater than 1:1 should raise concern for RV dysfunction.[27] It is also in the short axis that the "D-sign" can be seen. The D-sign is a flattening of the normal curvature of the interventricular septum giving the LV a "D" shape. As pressures in the RV increase, the D-sign will impose on the LV throughout a longer portion of the cardiac cycle. Elevated pressures and septal bowing lead to decreased LV filling and can contribute to a component of cardiogenic shock. Care must be taken to ensure images are taken as perpendicular to the long axis as possible, as off-axis views may falsely seems to represent a D-sign.

The apical four-chamber view may offer confirmation of the above findings but also offers additional insight into RV function. It is in the four-chamber view that a tricuspid annular plane systolic excursion (TAPSE) can be measured as well as identification "McConnell's sign." The TAPSE is a linear measurement of RV function that has shown good inter-reliability[28] and prognosis in confirmed PE.[29–32] Its measurement is obtained using the M-mode function, placing the line of measurement through the lateral annulus of the tricuspid valve. The longitudinal displacement of the tricuspid annulus is measured at its peak during systole to the through during diastole. An abnormal cutoff value is less than 17 to 18 mm and a value of less than 15 mm has been shown to predict 30-day mortality.[31]

The four-chamber view is also useful for identifying a right heart strain pattern known as the "McConnell's sign." This sign comprises hypokinesis of the right ventricular free wall with preservation of the apex.[27] Initially thought to be a highly specific finding for acute PE, these abnormal dynamics can occur with other acute right heart pathology. McConnell and colleagues[33] discussed this finding in their 1996 publication and reported a high specificity of 0.94 for acute PE with a negative predictive value of 0.96. This study included 126 patients with right ventricular dysfunction and suggested that this echocardiographic finding should "raise the level of clinical suspicion for the diagnosis of acute PE." Since 1996, numerous studies have been published attempting to reproduce the original findings; however, not all have been congruent. Subsequent studies have shown that COPD exacerbations and RV infarcts may also produce a McConnell's sign questioning its broad application. More recently, Dwyer and colleagues published a prospective study in 2017, limiting inclusion criteria to those with suspected or imaging confirmed acute pulmonary emboli. The authors reported a specificity of 0.98 and a sensitivity of 0.22.[34] This study suggests that in cases where there is a high suspicion for acute PE, McConnell's sign may be useful as a means to support further imaging, diagnosis, and definitive management.

Additional more advanced echo techniques include the measurement of tricuspid regurgitation and calculation of right ventricular systolic pressures, right ventricular stroke volume assessment, right ventricular outflow pattern assessment, and pulmonary artery acceleration time measurement. These techniques may offer further insight into the prognosis and diagnosis of PE but are beyond the scope of this text. It is worth noting that many pathologies can cause acute RV dysfunction and bedside ultrasound is insufficiently sensitive or specific for confirming the diagnosis. Identifying the presence of proximal DVTs can further support the diagnosis of PE as the cause of acute cor pulmonale findings seen on bedside echocardiography. Lack of right ventricular dilatation, lack of intraventricular septal dyskinesia, and lack of a depressed TAPSE on bedside echocardiography decrease the likelihood of finding a massive pulmonary embolus.

BEDSIDE TRANSESOPHAGEAL ECHOCARDIOGRAPHY

Performing a bedside transesophageal echocardiogram is an emerging technique for diagnosing PE as the cause of extreme shock or cardiac arrest. Performing this imaging technique in the emergency department requires an intubated patient along with additional training and equipment but can quickly identify massive PEs such as saddle PEs or in the proximal main branches.

CT PULMONARY ANGIOGRAPHY

CT pulmonary angiography (CTPA) is the gold standard for identifying the presence of an acute PE. It is both sensitive and specific and can assess the degree and severity of the anatomic clot burden. The decision to proceed with a contrast and radiation load during the workup of a potential PE is a frequent quandary ubiquitous in emergency medicine. The radiation load is of legitimate concern and CTPA is not indicated in the low-risk population, especially those with a negative d-dimer. Some populations, such as the elderly or pregnant, preclude the use of d-dimer and CTPA may become increasingly necessary in these populations to satisfactorily exclude the diagnosis of PE. The one major shortcoming of CTPA is its inability to accurately identify chronic thromboembolic PEs, which are better identified on ventilation–perfusion scintigraphy (V/Q scan).

VENTILATION–PERFUSION SCINTIGRAPHY

V/Q scan can be used when CTPA is unavailable, in patients who cannot receive contrast or when assessing for chronic PE. Ventilation–perfusion scintigraphy involves two image collection phases. In one phase, the patient inhales a radioactive gas showing ventilation, followed by a second phase with the injection of a radiopharmaceutical showing perfusion. These two images are overlapped and compared with identify mismatch. The injected radiopharmaceutical eventually collects in the urinary system, adjacent to the female reproductive organs, which makes this form of testing unsuitable for use in pregnant patients.

RISK STRATIFICATION

Given the wide range of clinical presentation of PE, the emergency physician must be well versed in risk stratification. Identifying which patients are safe for discharge versus those that will require a higher level of care can be challenging. The safety of discharge largely relies of vital signs, cardiac markers, and evidence of right heart strain whether by echocardiography or CT imaging. Two commonly deployed decision-making tools are the pulmonary embolism severity index (PESI) and the simplified PESI. The PESI score uses 11 clinical findings to risk stratify patients into five classes. Class I represents a 0% to 1.6% 30-day risk of mortality, whereas Class V represents 10% to 24.5%.[35] The sPESI score involves six dichotomous clinical findings when negative identify patients safe for discharge.[36] Both have been validated in several studies.[37,38] Incorporated in the sPESI score is heart rate greater than 110 bpm and SBP less than 100 mm Hg, which reaffirms the value of the shock index in patients with PE.

Cardiac enzymes including the troponin and pro-brain natriuretic peptide are useful in risk stratification. In normotensive patients ultimately identified to have right ventricular strain by echocardiography or CT imaging, the pro-BNP has been shown to have a sensitivity of 88% to 90% and a specificity of 68% to 75%. Alternatively, the troponin has shown a 62% to 82% sensitivity and 78% to 93% specificity.[39,40] In a meta-analysis, an elevated troponin was associated with both short-term mortality (OR

5.2) and risk of death (OR 9.4) secondary to PE. This risk was also shown in hemodynamically stable patients (OR 5.4).[41]

Presence or absence of lower extremity venous clot burden has also been investigated with outcomes in PE. Approximately half of the patients presenting with PE will have concomitant lower extremity thrombosis. Results of studies identifying correlation between DVT and mortality have been mixed; from no association[34] to a recent meta-analysis demonstrating an OR of 1.9.[42]

Presence of right ventricular dysfunction whether diagnosed by CT or echocardiography should always raise concern for short-term mortality and morbidity and warrants admission with possible intervention. Further discussion of echocardiography and CT imaging in PE is discussed below.

MANAGEMENT OF THE MASSIVE PULMONARY EMBOLISM

There are multiple treatment options for massive PE making it difficult for emergency clinicians to quickly identify the best treatments that are available in their institution. Therefore, guidelines recommend that a team-based approach be used to manage massive PE. This has led to the creation of a multidisciplinary team called PE response teams or PERT at many hospitals.

Initial resuscitation should include standard supportive therapy with the understanding that the critically ill PE patient has very little preload reserve. Initially, fluid resuscitation may improve vitals by supporting preload, however, the extent at which fluids benefit hemodynamics is unknown. Although no high-quality data exist on appropriate fluid resuscitation in right ventricular failure, experimental models have shown the deleterious effects of fluids when compared with inotropes.[43] Clinicians should be careful to avoid the so-called "PE death spiral" encountered when the pressures in the RV become elevated enough to push the interventricular septum into the LV, decreasing the LVEDV. With a fixed ejection fraction, reduction in LVEDV will continually decrease stroke volume causing cardiac output to become further compromised eventually leading to circulatory collapse.[44]

Intubation of a patient with right heart failure is tenuous in a best-case scenario. Owing to the RVs inability to tolerate changes in pressure, intubation can characteristically be challenging. Intubation and subsequent positive pressure ventilation will decrease RV preload as well as increase RV afterload, challenging cardiac output further.[44] There is no accepted universal approach to intubation, regarding medications, awake versus rapid sequence, or other factors; however, having a well-strategized, team approach is prudent. After intubation, minimizing pressures or tidal volumes may minimize hemodynamic changes until stability is assured.[44]

In the setting of cardiac arrest or the peri-arrest state, systemic thrombolysis should be attempted. A half dose protocol has been widely suggested that using a 50 mg IV bolus is just as efficacious but with a lower complication rate than the traditional 100 mg bolus,[45] a meta-analysis later supported this finding.[46] However, a more recent observational cohort study of 420 hospitals over 5 years with 699 patients receiving low-dose rtPA and 3069 receiving standard-dose rtPA found similar rates of complications with increased rates of treatment escalation in the low-dose group.[47] Given this conflicting data, it may be reasonable to stay with standard-dose rtPA in most situations and limit low-dose rtPA to patients with increased risk of bleeding (pregnant, elderly, small, or with another condition lending them to a high risk of bleeding).

Surgical thrombectomy, or pulmonary embolectomy, was the earliest treatment attempted for massive PE. The first attempt pulmonary embolectomy was performed by Friedrich Trendelenburg in 1908. It was performed without the use of a bypass machine and unfortunately the patient bled to death in the operating room.[48] The need for extracorporeal circulation inspired John Gibbon to develop cardiopulmonary bypass during his care of a patient with massive PE in 1931.[49] With the advent of heparin, pulmonary embolectomy on bypass pump became the mainstay of treatment of PE, until thrombolytics were introduced in the 1970s when surgical pulmonary embolectomy started to become considered obsolete due to the risk of critical hemorrhage.

The use of extracorporeal membrane oxygenation (ECMO) in the OR led to its use outside the OR as well for critical patients crashing from obstructive shock. The blockage being in the pulmonary artery necessitates the need for the veno-arterial (VA) ECMO rather than venovenous ECMO. Survival from massive PE on VA ECMO has been reported as high as 74%.[50] The same group found that greater than 30 minutes of CPR before initiation of VA ECMO led to only a 10% survival. The ARREST trial, a 2020 study of out-of-hospital cardiac arrest, not specific to PE, found survival to hospital discharge with standard ACLS to be 7% (1.6–30.2) versus 43% (21.3–67.7) in the ECMO-facilitated resuscitation group.[51] These results are promising but the real-world applicability of this study to the care of massive PE is uncertain and further study remains to be done.

MANAGEMENT OF SUBMASSIVE PULMONARY EMBOLISM

The management of submassive PE is controversial and likely varies based on local practices. The question as to whether catheter-directed therapy versus anticoagulation alone versus systemic thrombolysis remains debated with no definitive conclusion.

Catheter-directed therapy has been a method suggested to potentially reduce the systemic rtPA load while maintaining its effectiveness by applying it directly to the thrombus. CDT is typically performed by an interventional cardiologist or interventional radiologist. A catheter is placed through a large vein and the catheter is directed to the site of thrombosis, usually in the main pulmonary artery or one of its branches. Although in theory, CDT is a logical route to reduce exposure to systemic rtPA, studies have shown mixed results and have been heavily scrutinized.

The landmark SEATTLE II trial evaluated both intermediate- and high-risk patients with PE. This prospective study of 150 patients showed a reduction in RV end-diastolic diameter and a substantial decrease in mean pulmonary arterial pressure.[52] Both endpoints were achieved without any patients suffering from intracranial hemorrhage. Similarly, a single-site study of 106 patients with intermediate-risk PE confirmed the safety and efficacy of RV dilation reduction but was not randomized to systemic thrombolysis or anticoagulation alone.[53]

Although these studies are promising, other studies have not shown similar results. A retrospective study of 268 patients with submassive pulmonary emboli failed to show a mortality difference or difference in rates of ICH.[54] Another retrospective study of 1915 patients did not show any difference in ICH but paradoxically showed a significant increase in bleeding (16.0 vs 8.7%; $P < .001$) with CDT, whereas in-hospital mortality was lower (6.5 vs 10.0%; $P = .02$) in the CDT arm.[55] It is worth noting that these studies are often criticized for patient selection bias, being performed at single centers, influenced by local practices, and lack of a control group. For these reasons, larger, multicenter prospective studies are still needed. Currently, the CHEST 2016 and European 2019 guidelines both recommend systemic rtPA over CDT.[56,57]

MANAGEMENT OF SUBSEGMENTAL PULMONARY EMBOLISM

A specific area of controversy in the treatment of PE lies in the management of the SSPE. The 2016 CHEST update antithrombotic guidelines suggested, "In patients with SSPE (no involvement of more proximal pulmonary arteries) and no proximal DVT in the legs, who have a low risk for recurrent VTE (see text), we suggest clinical surveillance over anticoagulation (Grade 2C)."[56] There are no prospective randomized trials, and there is sharply conflicting evidence of lesser quality data analysis, leading to a strong disagreement among experts. The most often cited study to support nontreatment had 79 SSPEs but only nine patients were in the nontreatment group.[58] In contrast, a post hoc review of 3728 patients showed that SSPE carried a significantly higher risk of recurrent VTE compared with the non-PE group with a hazard ratio of 3.8.[59] In fact, there was no statistical difference in the risk of both recurrence and mortality in SSPE compared with larger PEs. When a clinical scenario of SSPE was presented to 183 specialists of varied backgrounds who treat PE, in the absence of cancer 72% of physicians would choose to treat.[60]

Owing to the prevalence of conflicting low-quality evidence and a dearth of high-quality evidence, most guidelines and experts recommend using an individualized and shared decision-making approach to anticoagulation of SSPE.

LOW-RISK PULMONARY EMBOLISM AND LONG-TERM ANTICOAGULATION

For patients diagnosed with pulmonary emboli but are deemed to be low-risk, initiation of oral anticoagulation from the emergency department is considered the mainstay of management. Parenteral anticoagulation or vitamin K antagonists can be considered; however, given the efficacy of direct oral anticoagulants (DOACs), these may be preferred. DOACs work by inhibiting a single component of the coagulation cascade; thrombin for dabigatran and Factor Xa for rivaroxaban and apixaban. These agents have fairly stable pharmacokinetics, oral availability, and do not require therapeutic level monitoring. Furthermore, meta-analysis has shown non-inferiority when compared with VKAs in preventing negative outcomes in DVTs and actually showed lower bleeding complication rates.[61] DOACs safety and efficacy in treating atrial fibrillation, left ventricular thrombi, and deep venous thrombosis have led to its adoption in the treatment of PE.[57]

Recent studies have shown good safety and efficacy with the reduced dose, long-term anticoagulation for the prevention of recurrent VTE.[62–64] It remains to be determined whether reduced dose, long-term anticoagulation can reduce long-term mortality rates in preventing recurrent PE.

Unprovoked or recurrent PE should be worked up for the presence of clotting disorders and treated with long-term anticoagulation. These include disorders such as Factor V Leiden disorder, deficiency of protein C or S and antiphospholipid syndrome. However, provoked PE can be treated with a shorter duration of anticoagulation.

CLINICAL OUTCOMES

Long-term clinical outcomes from PE are strongly correlated with initial clinical severity as well as the time to diagnosis and treatment. Massive PE has significantly worse survival despite treatment than low-risk PE, as would be expected.

In one contemporary study, overall long-term mortality was 40.1% with a median follow-up length of approximately 4 years. When stratified into massive, high-risk, and low-risk severity PEs, overall mortality in each group was 71.4%, 44.5%, and 28.1%, respectively. Short-term mortality was 57.1%, 6.7%, and 3.5%, respectively, as well. These results highlight both the immediate severity of massive PE as well as the nonzero mortality associated with low-risk PE. Although the thromboembolic event itself was the leading short-term (less than 30-day) cause of death, long-term (greater than 30 days) cause of death was more associated with underlying conditions such as malignancy, cardiac, or respiratory disease, with PE being listed as the fourth leading attributable cause of long-term mortality.[65]

When left untreated overall mortality for PE is 30%. Risk for recurrent VTE and PE is more closely related to the underlying cause and whether the thromboembolic event was provoked or unprovoked. The current recommendation is to continue long-term anticoagulation in the setting of unprovoked thromboembolic events. Overall the risk of recurrent VTE is 20% to 30% over 5 years[2,3] and was the cause of long-term deaths in 7% of patients.[65–67]

CTEPH is a rare but serious long-term complication leading to pulmonary hypertension. CTEPH can occur some time after a silent PE or after one that was inadequately or ineffectively treated. This can lead to significant morbidity if left undiagnosed and can easily be missed on standard CT angiography. There have been suggestions for 3-month follow-up clinical examination, echocardiography, angiography, or V/Q scans to ensure treatment success after acute PE. It remains to be determined what the best follow-up would be, if any, and if it would lead to improved outcomes. Currently, the preferred treatment of CTEPH is pulmonary endarterectomy (PEA) and tends to have significantly improved long-term morbidity with a relative death reduction rate of 63% compared with other therapies.[68] Patients' status post-PEA carries a significantly better prognosis than most other forms of pulmonary hypertension. Unfortunately, PEA is a technically complex surgery performed only at specialized centers, is not available for all patients, and carries an approximately 5% mortality.[69] For patients unable to receive PEA, balloon pulmonary angioplasty is an option shown to improve short-term hemodynamic parameters but has not been shown to improve long-term morbidity or mortality.[70]

SUMMARY

Diagnosis and management of pulmonary emboli are a crucial skill for any emergency physician. The wide range of clinical presentations and multiple modalities of testing and risk stratification exemplify the challenges in this population. Management of intermediate risk and high risk or massive pulmonary emboli still remains a target of research and debate. Identifying the resources and protocols at any particular institution is prudent given these practice variations.

CLINICS CARE POINTS

- Pulmonary embolism constitutes a significant burden of disease in both the outpatient and inpatient settings.
- Clinical presentation can widely vary, being familiar with risk factors and clinical decision-making tools can assist in workup.
- Management of the patient with a pulmonary emboli should focus on ensuring initial hemodynamic stability.
- Guidelines recommend treatment with thrombolytics in the setting of hemodynamic instability; however, there is an ongoing debate to the proper management of submassive pulmonary embolism.

REFERENCES

1. Pollack CV, et al. Clinical characteristics, management, and outcomes of patients diagnosed with acute pulmonary embolism in the emergency department: initial

report of EMPEROR (Multicenter Emergency Medicine Pulmonary Embolism in the Real World Registry). J Am Coll Cardiol 2011;57(6):700–6.

2. Anderson FA Jr, et al. Estimated annual numbers of US acute-care hospital patients at risk for venous thromboembolism. Am J Hematol 2007;82(9):777–82.

3. Raskob GE, et al. Thrombosis: a major contributor to global disease burden. Arterioscler Thromb Vasc Biol 2014;34(11):2363–71.

4. Heit JA, et al. Incidence of venous thromboembolism in hospitalized patients vs community residents. Mayo Clin Proc 2001;76(11):1102–10.

5. Alikhan R, et al. Fatal pulmonary embolism in hospitalised patients: a necropsy review. J Clin Pathol 2004;57(12):1254–7.

6. van Langevelde K, et al. Finding the origin of pulmonary emboli with a total-body magnetic resonance direct thrombus imaging technique. Haematologica 2013; 98(2):309–15.

7. van Dam LF, et al. Clinical and computed tomography characteristics of COVID-19 associated acute pulmonary embolism: a different phenotype of thrombotic disease? Thromb Res 2020;193:86–9.

8. Rose PS, Punjabi NM, Pearse DB. Treatment of right heart thromboemboli. Chest 2002;121(3):806–14.

9. Morrone D, Morrone V. Acute pulmonary embolism: focus on the clinical picture. Korean Circ J 2018;48(5):365–81.

10. Bougouin W, et al. Pulmonary embolism related sudden cardiac arrest admitted alive at hospital: management and outcomes. Resuscitation 2017;115:135–40.

11. Bougouin W, et al. Factors associated with pulmonary embolism-related sudden cardiac arrest. Circulation 2016;134(25):2125–7.

12. Keller K, et al. Typical symptoms for prediction of outcome and risk stratification in acute pulmonary embolism. Int Angiol 2016;35(2):184–91.

13. Keller K, et al. Evaluation of risk stratification markers and models in acute pulmonary embolism: rationale and design of the MARS-PE (Mainz Retrospective Study of Pulmonary Embolism) study programme. Acta Medica (Hradec Kralove) 2018; 61(3):93–7.

14. Duplyakov D, et al. Value of syncope in patients with high-to-intermediate risk pulmonary artery embolism. Eur Heart J Acute Cardiovasc Care 2015;4(4):353–8.

15. Thomson D, et al. ECG in suspected pulmonary embolism. Postgrad Med J 2019; 95(1119):12–7.

16. Ferrari E, et al. The ECG in pulmonary embolism. Predictive value of negative T waves in precordial leads–80 case reports. Chest 1997;111(3):537–43.

17. Digby GC, et al. The value of electrocardiographic abnormalities in the prognosis of pulmonary embolism: a consensus paper. Ann Noninvasive Electrocardiol 2015;20(3):207–23.

18. Kline JA, et al. Prospective multicenter evaluation of the pulmonary embolism rule-out criteria. J Thromb Haemost 2008;6(5):772–80.

19. Kline JA, et al. Clinical criteria to prevent unnecessary diagnostic testing in emergency department patients with suspected pulmonary embolism. J Thromb Haemost 2004;2(8):1247–55.

20. Wolf SJ, et al. Prospective validation of Wells Criteria in the evaluation of patients with suspected pulmonary embolism. Ann Emerg Med 2004;44(5):503–10.

21. Wells PS, et al. Excluding pulmonary embolism at the bedside without diagnostic imaging: management of patients with suspected pulmonary embolism presenting to the emergency department by using a simple clinical model and d-dimer. Ann Intern Med 2001;135(2):98–107.

22. Schouten HJ, et al. Diagnostic accuracy of conventional or age adjusted D-dimer cut-off values in older patients with suspected venous thromboembolism: systematic review and meta-analysis. BMJ 2013;346:f2492.
23. Righini M, et al. Age-adjusted D-dimer cutoff levels to rule out pulmonary embolism: the ADJUST-PE study. JAMA 2014;311(11):1117–24.
24. Sharp AL, et al. An age-adjusted d-dimer threshold for emergency department patients with suspected pulmonary embolus: accuracy and clinical implications. Ann Emerg Med 2016;67(2):249–57.
25. van der Hulle T, et al. Simplified diagnostic management of suspected pulmonary embolism (the YEARS study): a prospective, multicentre, cohort study. Lancet 2017;390(10091):289–97.
26. Kabrhel C, et al. Multicenter Evaluation of the YEARS Criteria in Emergency Department Patients Evaluated for Pulmonary Embolism. Acad Emerg Med 2018;25(9):987–94.
27. Rudski LG, et al. Guidelines for the echocardiographic assessment of the right heart in adults: a report from the American Society of Echocardiography endorsed by the European Association of Echocardiography, a registered branch of the European Society of Cardiology, and the Canadian Society of Echocardiography. J Am Soc Echocardiogr 2010;23(7):685–713, quiz 786-8.
28. Kopecna D, et al. Interobserver reliability of echocardiography for prognostication of normotensive patients with pulmonary embolism. Cardiovasc Ultrasound 2014;12:29.
29. Paczynska M, et al. Tricuspid annulus plane systolic excursion (TAPSE) has superior predictive value compared to right ventricular to left ventricular ratio in normotensive patients with acute pulmonary embolism. Arch Med Sci 2016; 12(5):1008–14.
30. Daley J, et al. Emergency physician performed tricuspid annular plane systolic excursion in the evaluation of suspected pulmonary embolism. Am J Emerg Med 2017;35(1):106–11.
31. Lobo JL, et al. Prognostic significance of tricuspid annular displacement in normotensive patients with acute symptomatic pulmonary embolism. J Thromb Haemost 2014;12(7):1020–7.
32. Alerhand S, Hickey SM. Tricuspid Annular Plane Systolic Excursion (TAPSE) for Risk Stratification and Prognostication of Patients with Pulmonary Embolism. J Emerg Med 2020;58(3):449–56.
33. McConnell MV, et al. Regional right ventricular dysfunction detected by echocardiography in acute pulmonary embolism. Am J Cardiol 1996;78(4):469–73.
34. Dwyer KH, Rempell JS, Stone MB. Diagnosing centrally located pulmonary embolisms in the emergency department using point-of-care ultrasound. Am J Emerg Med 2018;36(7):1145–50.
35. Aujesky D, et al. Derivation and validation of a prognostic model for pulmonary embolism. Am J Respir Crit Care Med 2005;172(8):1041–6.
36. Jimenez D, et al. Simplification of the pulmonary embolism severity index for prognostication in patients with acute symptomatic pulmonary embolism. Arch Intern Med 2010;170(15):1383–9.
37. Donze J, et al. Prospective validation of the Pulmonary Embolism Severity Index. A clinical prognostic model for pulmonary embolism. Thromb Haemost 2008; 100(5):943–8.
38. Zhou XY, et al. The prognostic value of pulmonary embolism severity index in acute pulmonary embolism: a meta-analysis. Respir Res 2012;13:111.

39. Choi HS, et al. Usefulness of cardiac biomarkers in the prediction of right ventricular dysfunction before echocardiography in acute pulmonary embolism. J Cardiol 2012;60(6):508–13.

40. Weekes AJ, et al. Diagnostic accuracy of right ventricular dysfunction markers in normotensive emergency department patients with acute pulmonary embolism. Ann Emerg Med 2016;68(3):277–91.

41. Becattini C, Vedovati MC, Agnelli G. Prognostic value of troponins in acute pulmonary embolism: a meta-analysis. Circulation 2007;116(4):427–33.

42. Becattini C, et al. Risk stratification of patients with acute symptomatic pulmonary embolism based on presence or absence of lower extremity DVT: systematic review and meta-analysis. Chest 2016;149(1):192–200.

43. Ghignone M, Girling L, Prewitt RM. Volume expansion versus norepinephrine in treatment of a low cardiac output complicating an acute increase in right ventricular afterload in dogs. Anesthesiology 1984;60(2):132–5.

44. Wanner PM, Filipovic M. The right ventricle-you may forget it, but it will not forget you. J Clin Med 2020;9(2):432.

45. Wang C, et al. Efficacy and safety of low dose recombinant tissue-type plasminogen activator for the treatment of acute pulmonary thromboembolism: a randomized, multicenter, controlled trial. Chest 2010;137(2):254–62.

46. Zhang Z, et al. Lower dosage of recombinant tissue-type plasminogen activator (rt-PA) in the treatment of acute pulmonary embolism: a systematic review and meta-analysis. Thromb Res 2014;133(3):357–63.

47. Kiser TH, et al. Half-Dose Versus Full-Dose Alteplase for Treatment of Pulmonary Embolism. Crit Care Med 2018;46(10):1617–25.

48. Meyer JA. Friedrich Trendelenburg and the surgical approach to massive pulmonary embolism. Arch Surg 1990;125(9):1202–5.

49. Gibbon JH Jr. The development of the heart-lung apparatus. Rev Surg 1970;27(4):231–44.

50. Sakuma M, et al. Percutaneous cardiopulmonary support for the treatment of acute pulmonary embolism: summarized review of the literature in Japan including our own experience. Ann Vasc Dis 2009;2(1):7–16.

51. Yannopoulos D, et al. Advanced reperfusion strategies for patients with out-of-hospital cardiac arrest and refractory ventricular fibrillation (ARREST): a phase 2, single centre, open-label, randomised controlled trial. Lancet 2020;396(10265):1807–16.

52. Piazza G, et al. A Prospective, Single-Arm, Multicenter Trial of Ultrasound-Facilitated, Catheter-Directed, Low-Dose Fibrinolysis for Acute Massive and Submassive Pulmonary Embolism: The SEATTLE II Study. JACC Cardiovasc Interv 2015;8(10):1382–92.

53. Tu T, et al. A Prospective, Single-Arm, Multicenter Trial of Catheter-Directed Mechanical Thrombectomy for Intermediate-Risk Acute Pulmonary Embolism: The FLARE Study. JACC Cardiovasc Interv 2019;12(9):859–69.

54. Bloomer TL, et al. Safety of catheter-directed thrombolysis for massive and submassive pulmonary embolism: Results of a multicenter registry and meta-analysis. Catheter Cardiovasc Interv 2017;89(4):754–60.

55. Geller BJ, et al. Outcomes of catheter-directed versus systemic thrombolysis for the treatment of pulmonary embolism: A real-world analysis of national administrative claims. Vasc Med 2020;25(4):334–40.

56. Kearon C, et al. Antithrombotic Therapy for VTE Disease: CHEST Guideline and Expert Panel Report. Chest 2016;149(2):315–52.

57. Konstantinides SV, et al. 2019 ESC Guidelines for the diagnosis and management of acute pulmonary embolism developed in collaboration with the European Respiratory Society (ERS): The Task Force for the diagnosis and management of acute pulmonary embolism of the European Society of Cardiology (ESC). Eur Respir J 2019;54(3):1901647.

58. Raslan IA, et al. Rates of Overtreatment and Treatment-Related Adverse Effects Among Patients With Subsegmental Pulmonary Embolism. JAMA Intern Med 2018;178(9):1272–4.

59. den Exter PL, et al. Risk profile and clinical outcome of symptomatic subsegmental acute pulmonary embolism. Blood 2013;122(7):1144–9, quiz 1329.

60. den Exter PL, et al. Physicians' management approach to an incidental pulmonary embolism: an international survey. J Thromb Haemost 2013;11(1):208–13.

61. van der Hulle T, et al. Effectiveness and safety of novel oral anticoagulants as compared with vitamin K antagonists in the treatment of acute symptomatic venous thromboembolism: a systematic review and meta-analysis. J Thromb Haemost 2014;12(3):320–8.

62. Agnelli G, et al. Apixaban for extended treatment of venous thromboembolism. N Engl J Med 2013;368(8):699–708.

63. Investigators E, et al. Oral rivaroxaban for symptomatic venous thromboembolism. N Engl J Med 2010;363(26):2499–510.

64. Weitz JI, et al. Rivaroxaban or Aspirin for Extended Treatment of Venous Thromboembolism. N Engl J Med 2017;376(13):1211–22.

65. Gupta R, et al. Long-term mortality after massive, submassive, and low-risk pulmonary embolism. Vasc Med 2020;25(2):141–9.

66. Eichinger S, et al. Risk assessment of recurrence in patients with unprovoked deep vein thrombosis or pulmonary embolism: the Vienna prediction model. Circulation 2010;121(14):1630–6.

67. Couturaud F, et al. Six Months vs Extended Oral Anticoagulation After a First Episode of Pulmonary Embolism: the PADIS-PE Randomized Clinical Trial. JAMA 2015;314(1):31–40.

68. Delcroix M, et al. Long-term outcome of patients with chronic thromboembolic pulmonary hypertension: results from an international prospective registry. Circulation 2016;133(9):859–71.

69. Vistarini N, et al. Pulmonary endarterectomy in the elderly: safety, efficacy and risk factors. J Cardiovasc Med (Hagerstown) 2016;17(2):144–51.

70. Ogawa A, et al. Balloon pulmonary angioplasty for chronic thromboembolic pulmonary hypertension: results of a multicenter registry. Circ Cardiovasc Qual Outcomes 2017;10(11):e004029.

Special Procedures for Pulmonary Disease in the Emergency Department

Brian C. Park, MD[a], Haney Mallemat, MD[b]

KEYWORDS

- Thoracentesis • Chest tube thoracostomy • Pneumothorax • Pleural effusion
- Tracheostomy emergency • Fiberoptic intubation

KEY POINTS

- In the setting of pleural pathologies such as pleural effusions, hemothorax, and pneumothorax, thoracentesis, small- and large-bore chest tube thoracostomy are crucial skills to master for the emergency department (ED) physician.
- Management of tracheostomy emergencies, namely tube obstruction, dislodgement, or decannulation, requires a solid understanding of tracheostomy anatomy and a practiced algorithmic approach.
- Fiberoptic intubation is an essential skill in the ED; however, it is infrequently used and requires prior planning, preparation, and practice.

ACCESSING THE PLEURAL SPACE: THORACENTESIS AND CHEST TUBE THORACOTOMY

Introduction

Diseases of the pleural space can range in severity from asymptomatic to life-threatening. The pleural space is normally a potential space that is under negative pressure, but when air or fluid accumulates it leads to compressive effects resulting in respiratory and hemodynamic compromise.

Nature of the Problem/Diagnosis

Anatomy of the pleural space

The thoracic cavity is lined by thin serous membranes, or pleurae, which envelop a small potential space. The apposing pleurae consist of the visceral and parietal layers;

[a] Critical Care Medicine Program, Cooper Medical School of Rowan University, Cooper University Hospital, 1 Cooper Plaza, Dorrance 4th Floor, Suite D427, Camden, NJ 08103, USA;
[b] Emergency Medicine/Critical Care Medicine Program, Cooper Medical School of Rowan University, Cooper University Hospital, 1 Cooper Plaza, Dorrance 4th Floor, Suite D427, Camden, NJ 08103, USA
E-mail address: bpark05@gmail.com
Twitter: @CritCareNow (H.M.)

Emerg Med Clin N Am 40 (2022) 583–602
https://doi.org/10.1016/j.emc.2022.05.009
0733-8627/22/© 2022 Elsevier Inc. All rights reserved.

emed.theclinics.com

the visceral pleura wraps around the surface of the lung and invaginates into the interlobular fissures whereas the parietal pleura lines the chest wall, diaphragm, and mediastinum. The pleural space is normally under negative pressure to allow inflation of the lungs during inspiration; a reduction in this negative pressure may compromise inspiration and expiration.

The pleural space provides a lubricated interface that allows sliding of the lungs in relation to the chest wall. Normally, there is a physiologic amount of serous fluid in the pleural space to provide lubrication of the serosal surfaces during respiration; this amounts to about 0.26 mL/kg of body mass or about 7 to 16 mL of fluid.[1-3] There is a homeostasis in the normal pleural space between the influx of fluid and removal by the lymphatic system.

Pathophysiology of the pleural space
A pleural effusion is an abnormal amount of fluid in the pleural space. The most common causes of a pathophysiologic pleural effusion in adults are congestive heart failure, pneumonia, malignancy, pulmonary embolism, and cirrhosis.[4,5] In children, the most common cause is pneumonia.[6,7] It is important to distinguish the pleural effusion as a transudate or exudate to help narrow the differential diagnosis, which then directs management and therapy.[8] Thoracentesis is a procedure that can be both diagnostic and therapeutic for pleural effusions.

Transudative effusions are secondary to leakage of fluid across non-injured capillary beds due to increased intravascular hydrostatic pressure or by a decrease in intravascular oncotic pressure.[8] These effusions have low cellular and protein content and are typically straw-colored and serous. Congestive heart failure and cirrhosis are common causes of transudative effusions.

Exudative effusions are secondary to pleural inflammation causing pleural membrane permeability or obstruction of lymphatic flow. Exudative effusions are commonly caused by malignancy, pneumonia, and Pulmonary Embolism.

Transudative Effusions	Exudative Effusions
Heart failure	
	Empyema
Nephrotic syndrome	
	Hemothorax
Cirrhosis	
	Malignancy
Hypoalbuminemia	
	Esophageal rupture
	Chylothorax

Pneumothorax
A pneumothorax is caused by the introduction of air in the intrapleural space. This can occur due to penetrating external trauma and introducing air from outside the chest cavity. It can also be due to air introduced from within the chest cavity such as in a ruptured emphysematous bleb, progression of pneumomediastinum from compromised esophageal, or tracheal lumens. Iatrogenic injury can also lead to pneumothorax such as from thoracostomy or thoracentesis, subclavian or internal jugular venous cannulation, positive pressure ventilation, bronchoscopy with endobronchial ultrasound (US) biopsy, transthoracic biopsy, or a complication of cardiopulmonary resuscitation.

Spontaneous pneumothorax
Spontaneous pneumothorax can be classified as primary or secondary. Primary is classically defined as occurring without precipitating event or underlying lung disease. Secondary is caused by underlying lung diseases such as emphysema, cystic fibrosis,

lung malignancy and so forth. Spontaneous pneumothorax can further be categorized as symptomatic or asymptomatic, as some pneumothoraces are found incidentally and do not cause the patients any symptoms and were found during workup for another issue.[9]

Recent literature supports conservative management of spontaneous asymptomatic pneumothorax rather than procedural intervention as >90% of cases resolve spontaneously and with fewer recurrences.[5,10]

Tension pneumothorax is a life-threatening emergency that results in hemodynamic and respiratory compromise. One example is when air enters the pleural space through a flap-like defect in the pleura that acts like a one-way valve. Air enters the pleural space during inspiration but the pleural flap closes on expiration and air cannot exit. This is commonly seen in the emergency department (ED) due to penetrating thoracic trauma, but can also result as a complication of esophageal or tracheal injury, or due to positive pressure ventilation. Patients with pneumothorax who need to be placed on positive pressure ventilation are at higher risk of tension pneumothorax so these patients should be considered for a "prophylactic" chest tube.[4]

Hemothorax
Bleeding into the pleural space can be a complication of venous or arterial bleeding. Causes include penetrating chest trauma, anticoagulant medications, hematologic malignancies, and vascular rupture (eg, ruptured AVM). Treatment for hemothorax should include tube thoracostomy to relieve the acumination of blood in the pleural space. If the hemothorax is secondary to arterial bleeding, consultation with surgical or interventional radiology will likely be required.[11]

Empyema
An empyema occurs when pus from an infection collects within the pleural space.

Most cases of empyema are due to complications of parapneumonic effusions but also occur due to infection after thoracic surgery and even with intra-abdominal infection. As a delay in intervention can lead to evolution of the empyema, loculation formation within 12 to 24 h, and increased morbidity and mortality, timeliness of chest tube insertion is very important.[12–14]

Indications for chest tube drainage include a large parapneumonic effusion >10 mm thickness, multi-loculated effusion, or a pleural fluid aspiration sample that shows frank pus (cloudy appearance and leukocyte count > 50,000/mm^3), positive Gram stain, or pleural fluid pH less than 7.2.[15] Traditionally, large-bore chest tubes have been indicated in the drainage of empyemas; however, current literature suggests empyemas may be successfully treated with 8-F to 12-F pigtail catheters and positioning of the catheter in the most dependent part of the effusion.[4,15–17]

Thrombolysis for empyema
A loculated empyema typically requires a specialized approach best addressed by computed tomography (CT) scan or US-guided chest tube placement. This approach is often combined with thrombolysis or thoracoscopy. Use of intrapleural combination therapy with both a fibrinolytic agent and DNase can be considered as initial therapy and can reduce the requirement for surgical referral.[18,19] Consideration and administration of intrapleural fibrinolytic therapy should be guided by local specialists such as thoracic surgeons or interventional pulmonologists.

Hepatic hydrothorax
Hepatic hydrothorax is a diagnosis of exclusion characterized by a transudative effusion in a patient with portal hypertension. Although thoracentesis may be warranted

for diagnostic purposes, large-bore chest tube drainage of hepatic hydrothorax is discouraged due to the associated high morbidity and mortality[20]

Diagnosing abnormalities of pleural space and pre-procedural planning

Abnormalities of the pleural space can be made by various imaging modalities. Initial diagnostic test is usually chest radiography (CXR) as it is noninvasive, expedient, and inexpensive. Blunting of the costophrenic angle may be seen on CXR; however, the sensitivity of CXR for detecting pleural effusion depends on the volume of fluid present and patient positioning. Supine radiographic images can be misleading as they have poor sensitivity for pleural effusion compared with CT imaging or even compared with lateral imaging (**Figs. 1** and **2**). Supine CXR can typically reveal a pleural effusion of 200–250 mL in an upright PA but lateral radiograph is more sensitive and can show effusions as small as 50–75 mL (4) (**Fig. 3**). Confirmation with bedside US can confirm that the radiographic opacity is indeed a pleural-based fluid.

Bedside US can also be used as the initial diagnostic modality as it is more sensitive than CXR and can detect small effusions of only 5 mL.[8] US is also able to identify the type of effusions such as simple versus complex. It may also help distinguish fluid collections from solid pleural lesions such as lung tissue that is compressed and atelectatic within the pleural fluid (**Fig. 4**). Imaging with US can be used to delineate anatomic landmarks before thoracentesis or can be used for real-time guidance of the procedure.[21] Identifying a lung point by US is a highly specific sign of pneumothorax (**Fig. 5**). Most importantly, US-guided thoracentesis is associated with a lower rate of major complications such pneumothorax and hemothorax— 0.3% to 3%, compared with 14% to 30% for percussion guided technique.22–26

A thoracentesis can be performed for either diagnostic or therapeutic purposes. Indications for tube thoracostomy are listed in **Box 1**. A newly discovered effusion measuring more than 1 mm requires diagnostic thoracentesis unless there is already a clear etiology of the effusion and no evidence of infection in the pleural space. Typically as little as 30 to 50 cc of diagnostic fluid is sufficient for analysis. Therapeutic thoracentesis can be performed to relieve dyspnea associated with large effusions and commonly drains >1L of fluid. There are no absolute contraindications for thoracentesis include other than a lack of pleural effusion. Relative contraindications include an overlying cutaneous infection, coagulopathy (INR >1.6), and thrombocytopenia (platelets <50), pleurodesis, or pleural adhesions at the site of entry.

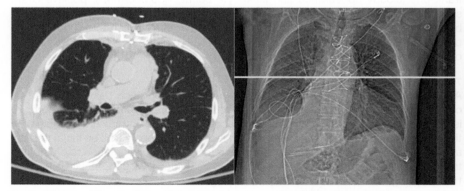

Fig. 1. CT scan of the chest showing a scout image on the right, although the patient is supine which does not reveal an obvious pleural effusion, but the corresponding axial image (at level of *yellow line*) on the left shows that there is a moderate right pleural effusion. This highlights the poor sensitivity of a supine image for the detection of pleural effusion.

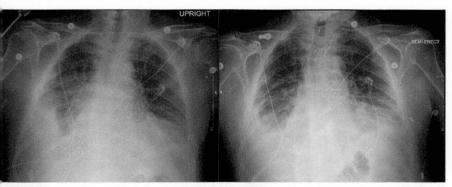

Fig. 2. Upright CXR (*left*) shows the right pleural effusion more clearly than the supine CXR (*right*).

A 30 to 50 cc pleural fluid sample should be obtained by thoracentesis for laboratory analysis and should be sent to the laboratory for analysis of pleural protein, lactate dehydrogenase, white blood cell count and differential, glucose, and pH. Other laboratory tests from the pleural sample should be guided by clinical suspicion and differential diagnosis (eg, in suspected esophageal rupture leading to pleural effusion, a salivary amylase should be detected in the pleural fluid).[27]

Contraindications
An absolute contraindication for chest tube thoracostomy is complete adherence of the lung to the chest wall.
Relative contraindications include coagulopathy, pulmonary adhesions from preexisting pulmonary structural disease, or skin infection over the insertion site.[28]

Chest Tube Size Selection
Pneumothorax or simple pleural effusion: small-sized bore 10 to 18 F. Smaller bore pleural catheters than 10 Fr are available in many hospitals, but these are easily kinked and should not be left in place to continue decompressing an unresolved pneumothorax.

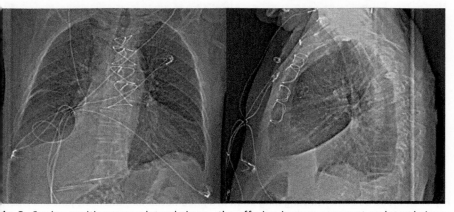

Fig. 3. Supine position versus lateral views—the effusion is more apparent on lateral views.

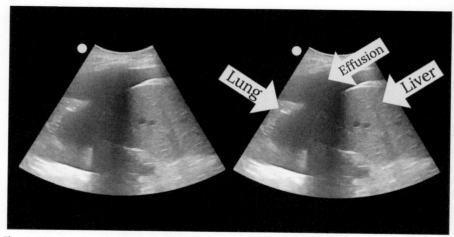

Fig. 4. Simple pleural effusion with compressive atelectatic lung.

Hemothorax or empyema: large-sized bore greater than 20 Fr has traditionally been used; however, recent literature suggests that there is no difference in failure rates comparing 14 Fr to 28 to 40 Fr in the setting of traumatic hemothorax.[29–32]

Patient Prep and Positioning

Thoracentesis for pleural effusion

1. Position the patient supine (**Fig. 6**A, B) or upright (**Fig. 6**C) based on patient compliance and location of the effusion after documenting informed consent for the procedure. Upright positioning is usually preferable for pleural effusion, and the patient can sit on the edge of the bed while leaning over a bedside table (see **Fig. 6**C).
2. Use US guidance to clearly locate the diaphragm with underlying liver or spleen and the overlying effusion. Identify the safest entry point based on the size and location of the effusion fluid pocket. Careful to avoid entry medial to the mid-scapular line

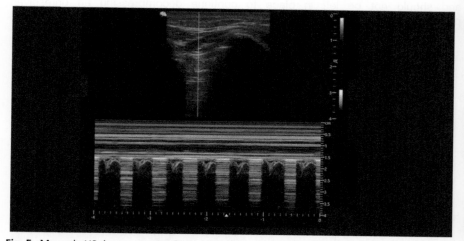

Fig. 5. M-mode US demonstrating lung point in a pneumothorax—this is the junction where lung sliding and absent lung sliding is seen.

Box 1
Indications for chest tube thoracostomy in trauma patients

Pneumothorax

Open: sucking chest wound
- Closed
- Simple
- Tension: after needle decompression
- In any mechanically ventilated patient

Hemothorax

Hemopneumothorax

Hemodynamically unstable patients with a chest-wall penetrating injury

Patients with penetrating chest trauma who are or could potentially be placed on mechanical

Ventilation

Recommended for patients with chest trauma who are going to be air-lifted and can potentially develop a pneumothorax.

---

because of the risk of injuring the aorta or intercostal arteries, which run more centrally and tortuously when it first enters the intercostal space at the spine.[8]
3. Follow sterile technique throughout the procedure to avoid the introduction of infection.

Procedural Approach

Thoracentesis for pleural effusion or chest tube for pneumothorax
Identify the entry point with ultrasound. Obtain thoracentesis kit or collect individual necessary components listed in **Fig. 7**

1. Sterilize and drape the skin
2. Anesthetize the skin, creating a skin wheal at the upper edge of the inferior rib using 1% or 2% lidocaine and a 25-gauge needle.
3. Use the upper edge of the inferior rib to minimize the risk of injury to the intercostal artery located along the inferior edge of the superior rib.

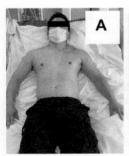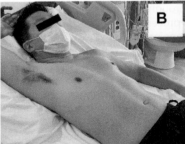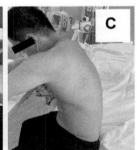

Fig. 6. (*A*) Anterior approach for small-bore chest tube for pneumothorax. (*B*) Anterior-lateral approach for small- or large-bore chest tube placement for pleural effusion/hemothorax/pneumothorax. (*C*) Upright and posterior-lateral positioning best suited for smaller effusions.

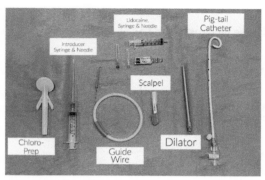

Fig 7. Equipment tray for small-bore chest tube placement for pneumothorax or for pleural effusion.

4. Using the same needle with lidocaine, position the needle at 90° to the skin at the upper edge of the inferior rib, and advance the needle depth while drawing negative pressure on the syringe plunger. If blood is aspirated, withdraw the needle and try another location within the same intercostal space.

5. If you hit bone with the needle tip, "walk" the needle tip superiorly over the rib and then continue advancing the needle depth through the intercostal space until the pleural space is entered. You may feel a change in the texture of the tissue and a "pop" may be felt.

6. Once in the pleural space, with the syringe plunger still under negative pressure, pleural fluid will start filling the syringe. If the procedure is for a pneumothorax, air will be aspirated into the syringe. Stop draining fluid/air, and grasp the needle at the skin to mark the proper depth of penetration needed. Inject a small amount of lidocaine to anesthetize the parietal pleura, and then slowly withdraw the needle while continuing to inject lidocaine to anesthetize the needle tract.

7. If no fluid/air is aspirated, the needle is likely too short.
   - If using a catheter-over needle approach, continue with step 9. If using the Seldinger approach, continue below with step 9b.

8. Attach the thoracentesis catheter to a 10-mL syringe.

9. Mark the depth of the pleural space on the thoracentesis catheter with your nondominant index finger and thumb that was determined from the anesthetic needle.

10. Advance the catheter through the anesthetized skin site and into the pleural space while drawing negative pressure with your dominant hand on the syringe plunger.

11. If there is difficulty advancing the needle–catheter unit at the skin surface, withdraw the needle–catheter unit, and use a scalpel to nick the skin to ease the entry of the needle–catheter unit through the skin.

12. When pleural fluid/air is aspirated, hold the depth of the needle steady with your dominant hand on the syringe, and using your nondominant hand twist the catheter to break its seal and then advance just the catheter (not the needle) into the pleural space.

13. Withdraw the needle and quickly attach a three-way stopcock to the catheter hub.

14. A 60-mL syringe can be used to aspirate fluid for diagnostic studies.

15. If performing a therapeutic thoracentesis, connect the three-way stopcock to the collection tubing. The other end of the collection tubing can be connected to a vacuum bottle or suction vacutainers in series.

6. If performing a small-bore chest tube see below. If only doing thoracentesis please go to step 18.

7. The recommended maximum of 1500 mL is to avoid symptomatic hypovolemia and reexpansion pulmonary edema. Larger volumes can be removed but this is not typically done in the ED.

8. Once done with fluid collection, have the patient perform a long exhale, and then withdraw the thoracentesis catheter.

9. Apply a pressure bandage with folded sterile gauze and silk tape.

20. Obtain a post-thoracentesis CXR.

Small-bore chest tube for pneumothorax or pleural effusion

9b. Once the skin, subcutaneous tissue, intercostal muscles, and pleura are anesthetized with the 25-gauge needle, use a larger 18-gauge needle to facilitate Seldinger wire entry.

10b. With a syringe attached, advance the Seldinger needle through the anesthetized tract while drawing negative pressure on the syringe. Once pleural fluid/air is withdrawn, advance the needle another 2 mm to ensure clearance of the needle bevel from the visceral pleura.

11b. Holding the needle depth steady, unscrew the syringe and introduce the Seldinger wire into the needle. Gently advance the wire which should thread smoothly. Any resistance is a sign that the wire is not in the pleural space, and the needle should be readjusted until the withdrawal of pleural fluid/air is again confirmed.

12b. With the wire threaded smoothly into the pleural cavity, withdraw the needle while maintaining the depth of the wire.

13b. Use a scalpel to make a 0.5-cm skin nick widening the wire entry hole.

14b. Advance the dilator over the wire and using a twisting motion carefully dilate the skin down through the pleura. Be careful to dilate in the direction of the wire and to "floss" the wire within the dilator to check that the wire is not kinked. Remove the dilator.

15b. Advance the small-bore chest tube over the wire until a depth of about 15–20 cm. Larger body habitus may require more depth. Remove the wire.

16b. Secure the chest tube to suction tubing.

17b. Suture the chest tube to the skin.

18b. Confirm the position of the chest tube with a CXR.

Large-bore tube thoracotomy

For hemothorax or empyema, large-bore tube sizing of 20 Fr or greater has traditionally been preferred to facilitate adequate drainage and minimize the risk of tube obstruction with clots or fibrinous exudate. However, as mentioned earlier, in traumatic hemothorax, recent evidence suggests that 14 Fr pigtail catheters compared with larger 28 to 40 Fr open chest tubes do have a difference in failure rates, but the smaller 14 Fr pigtail tube may be more comfortable and well tolerated by the patient.[29–32]

Another indication for blunt dissection chest tube thoracotomy is for a patient with large pneumothorax complicated by significant subcutaneous emphysema that obscures US evaluation of the pleural space. In this situation, blind entry of a needle into the pleural space is dangerous and can cause inadvertent damage to vital organs such as the spleen, liver, heart, and lung tissue itself. Blunt dissection with finger palpation offers a potentially safer technique than using the blind entry of a sharp instrument.

Chest Tube Thoracostomy Blunt Dissection Technique

1. Obtain a sterile surgical thoracotomy tray or collect individual necessary components as listed in **Fig. 8**. Large-bore chest tube will typically be 28–36 Fr.
2. Patient should be positioned supine. Expose the axilla by positioning the ipsilateral arm with the hand above and behind the head.
3. Identify the landmarks of the triangle of safety, which is bordered by the antero-lateral aspect of the latissimus dorsi, the lateral aspect of the pectoralis major, and a line drawn from the nipple intersecting the midaxillary line.
4. Administer IV sedation and analgesia.
5. Prep the area with iodine or chlorhexidine solution and apply sterile drapes.
6. Use a 25-gauge needle to infiltrate 2 to 3 mL of lidocaine in the incision site subcutaneously, and then infiltrate 5 to 10 mL of lidocaine into the subcutaneous tissue, intercostal muscles, and periosteum.
7. Remember to apply negative pressure on the syringe whenever advancing the depth; aspiration of blood or fluid can indicate the pleural space has been entered. Inject lidocaine into the pleural cavity and then withdraw the needle.
8. Use a scalpel to create a 3-cm incision parallel to the level of the fourth or fifth intercostal space midaxillary line. In obese patients with significant subcutaneous tissue, a larger incision of 3 to 5 cm may be necessary for the blunt dissection and to accommodate both finger and forceps entry to the pleural space.
9. Using round-tip forceps or a Kelly clamp, blunt dissect the subcutaneous tissue and muscle to create a tract from the incision site down to the intercostal space.
10. Do not remove the forceps, and use your index finger to palpate along the path of the forceps to the intercostal space. Blunt dissect further with the forceps as needed to adequately palpate the intercostal muscles and fascia with your index finger.
11. Position the closed tips of the forceps over the superior border of the rib and against the intercostal fascia/muscle. Using considerable force, advance the closed forceps until the pleura is punctured, and open and spread the instrument to separate the pleura and intercostal muscle tissue.
12. Do not remove the forceps until you can use your index finger to palpate the pleural space to confirm proper positioning.
13. Although your index finger secures the path into the pleural space, advance the chest tube into the pleural space using forceps clamped on the proximal end of the tube and introduce the tube until all the side holes are inside the pleural cavity. This is typically a depth of about 10 to 15 cm.

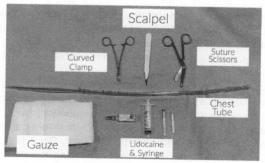

Fig. 8. Equipment tray for large-bore tube thoracostomy.

Table 1
Examples and rates of complications

Complications	Complication Rates
Pain	8%
Failure to place chest tube	2%
Hypotension	1.9%
Infection (skin or pleural space)	1.4%
Hemothorax	1.3%
Organ puncture	0.6%

Adapted from Ref.[33]

14. For a pneumothorax, direct the chest tube antero-apically. For hemothorax or empyema, direct the chest tube postero-basally.
15. Connect the tube to a chest drainage system; air bubbles will be seen in the fluid chamber if there is a pneumothorax, and blood/pus accumulation should be noted in the case of a hemothorax/empyema.
16. Use suture silk 1.0 to close the skin incision with the mattress technique and tie the loose ends around the tube to anchor it. Apply a sterile adhesive dressing.
17. Confirm the position of the chest tube with a CXR.

Complications

Complications have been reported with this procedure, which can generally be divided into insertional, positional, infectious, and technical involving the drainage system (**Table 1**). The most common complications are recurrent pneumothorax and chest tube misplacement.

A rare complication is re-expansion pulmonary edema reported at 0.6% of cases of chest tube drainage of pleural effusion.[33] Although the true clinical significance of re-expansion pulmonary edema is debated and many interventional pulmonologists routinely remove more than 1 L of pleural fluid, generally accepted practice in the ED is to limit the volume of pleural fluid removal to <1 to 1.5 L. Treatment is supportive.

Post-Procedure Care

Post-procedural imaging with CXR or bedside US is important not only to show proper positioning of the tube and improvement in the size of the pleural effusion but also to diagnose potential complications such as iatrogenic pneumothorax.

Discomfort at the site of thoracentesis is expected as the tube is a space-occupying device. Patients will typically feel less dyspnea immediately after the procedure if it is an acute process causing pleural effusion. Coughing is expected and normal as atelectatic lung tissue that was previously compressed by the effusion starts to re-expand. However, symptoms of life-threatening complications such as re-expansion pulmonary edema, iatrogenic hemothorax, or iatrogenic pneumothorax include chest discomfort, severe persistent cough, frothy sputum, dyspnea, tachypnea, tachycardia, and hypoxia.[34]

SUMMARY

ED thoracentesis and small- and large-bore chest tube thoracostomy are essential, potentially life-saving skills that the emergency physician should be proficient in performing. Thoracentesis can be performed to drain pleural fluid for diagnostic or therapeutic purposes. Small-bore chest tubes are typically inserted using the Seldinger technique for simple pleural effusions or pneumothoraces. We reserve large-bore chest tubes for hemothorax, empyema, or pneumothorax with extensive subcutaneous emphysema that precludes US guidance.

TRACHEOSTOMY EMERGENCIES
Introduction

Tracheostomy emergencies are uncommon but associated with significant morbidity and mortality. Emergency medicine providers should be familiar with the emergent management of tracheostomy emergencies, particularly obstructed tracheostomy and unplanned tracheostomy decannulation or dislodgment.

Nature of the Problem/Diagnosis

Tracheostomies can present unique airway challenges when presenting to the emergency room and emergency physicians must be adept in the initial management of complications related to tracheostomies. Most of the complications related to tracheostomies are minor and easily managed; however, 1% of tracheostomy patients will suffer a catastrophic complication for which mortality is very high.[35] Tube obstruction and tube dislodgement or decannulations are the life-threatening complications and the most feared complication in the ED.

Early tracheostomy complications are defined as occurring within 1 week of the tracheostomy placement and include bleeding (2%–5%), infection (−.5%), posterior membrane injury (rare), tracheostomy tube obstruction (3.5%), and early extubation (1%). Late complications occur more than 1-week post-procedure and are categorized anatomically. Suprastomal lesions include subglottic stenosis, tracheal stenosis, and granulation tissue formation. Stomal lesions typically result from fracture of the anterior tracheal wall during percutaneous dilational tracheostomy and in the anterior wall protruding into the tracheal lumen creating a fixed obstruction. Infrastomal complications include tracheal stenosis, tracheomalacia, tracheoesophageal fistula, and tracheoinnominate fistula.[36]

Tracheostomy versus laryngectomy

One important anatomic difference to keep in mind about tracheostomy compared with laryngectomy is that in a tracheostomy the upper airway is still potentially patent, whereas in a laryngectomy the trachea is open through the neck to the atmosphere without any connection to the upper airway. This point is particularly important in an emergency with a tracheostomy, as applying supplemental oxygen to the mouth and nose is important, and re-intubation from the upper airway is still a possibility. This is not the case with a laryngectomy.

Anatomy of a tracheostomy tube

The components of a tracheostomy tube are important to be familiar with, as shown in **Fig. 9**. The cuffed tracheostomy will have an attached pilot balloon and is designed to occlude the trachea to create a closed system completely without losing airway pressures up into the mouth. The outer cannula has a flange that allows the sutures or ties to secure the outer cannula down and in place. There is an inner cannula that should always be in place to catch secretions and should only be removed when suctioning the trach and for routine cleaning. The obturator is used to remove and replace the outer cannula.

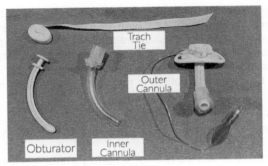

Fig. 9. Components of a tracheostomy tube.

Obstructed tracheostomy tube

Obstruction in the tracheostomy tube is a commonly encountered complication. A mucous plug within the inner cannula of the tracheostomy tube is usually the culprit, although bleeding, granulation tissue, and foreign objects can also cause obstruction.[35] Patients will present as mild dyspnea to overt respiratory distress. If patients are connected to a ventilator, peak pressures will be elevated due to the resistance created by the obstruction.

Treating obstruction

1. Remove the inner cannula. This maneuver by itself will often relieve the obstruction as mucous will be stuck in the inner cannula, but the remaining outer cannula is patent.
2. Pass a soft suction catheter through the remaining outer cannula and suction out any remaining debris.
3. Replace the inner cannula with a new, clean cannula.

Unplanned tube dislodgement or decannulation

In patient with a recently placed (<7 days) tracheostomy, a harrowing complication that can occur is an unplanned tracheostomy tube dislodgement or decannulation. This medical emergency of tube dislodgement occurs in approximately 1% of patients and mortality and morbidity is very high secondary to an inability to oxygenate or ventilate.[35–37] The absence of a mature tracheostomy tract in a recently placed tracheostomy can make replacement of the tracheostomy tube difficult and can lead to ventilation through a false tract. Factors predisposing to displacement include loose tracheostomy ties, neck edema, excess couching, airway edema, agitation, and poor placement of the tracheostomy.[38]

For a patient presenting to the ED with a displaced tracheostomy, first assess if the patient is in respiratory distress or not. If they are not in distress, determine when the tracheostomy was placed and how long before presentation did the decannulation occur. Even a mature stoma can narrow significantly in just a few hours making recannulation more difficult and may necessitate a smaller tracheostomy tube.[35] Replacement of the dislodged tracheostomy within 7 days of placement should be deferred when possible to the surgical team who placed the tracheostomy. If necessary by the emergency provider, replacement of this early tracheostomy should be attempted only with direct visualization with fiberoptic scope to prevent creating a false tract. Confirmation of proper placement can be performed with capnography (qualitative, quantitative, or waveform) or direct visualization with bronchoscopy if available.

McGrath et al proposed algorithms for the management of tracheostomy and laryngectomy airway emergencies in 2012.[37] There have been many adaptations based on these original algorithms, which can be tailored to best address the needs of different hospitals and departments based on their available resources and staff. The algorithm detailed below is our recommended pathway.

In the ED for a tracheostomy patient in respiratory distress, we use the following algorithm:

1. Apply oxygen to the patient's face and tracheostomy site
2. Emergent consult to a respiratory therapist and the otolaryngoscopy (ENT) service.
3. Call for emergency airway equipment including a new tracheostomy kit of the same size (and smaller) as well as a fiberoptic scope
4. Assess reason and date of tracheostomy placement
5. Remove inner cannula or speaking valve/cap
6. Pass soft suction catheter through outer cannula
   a. If the suction catheter passes easily and the obstruction is relieved
   b. Attach BVM and give two gentle breaths—if the chest wall rises with breaths and there is no evidence of subcutaneous emphysema, then the obstruction is relieved
7. If the suction catheter does not pass or if there is neck swelling indicating progressing subcutaneous emphysema with BVM ventilation, then STOP bagging and declare an emergency. This is a displaced tracheostomy.
8. Deflate the cuff. A partially displaced tracheostomy tube may with deflated cuff may allow airflow past the tracheostomy to the upper airways.
9. If the patient is stable: pass a slim bronchoscope through the tracheostomy to visualize the tracheal rings and confirm positioning. Avoid blinding inserting rigid objects such as a gum-elastic bougie as this can easily slip between tissue planes and create or exacerbate a false tract.
10. If the patient is unstable: deflate and remove the trach. Apply pressure with gauze to occlude the trach site.
11. Manage the airway via the mouth with non-rebreather or bag valve mask as you request advanced airway equipment to the bedside as well as drugs for rapid sequence intubation.
12. Perform orotracheal intubation and advance the ETT cuff past the trach site.
13. If reintubation from above is difficult or impossible, insert a finger into the trach site. Confirm your finger is in the trachea by palpating tracheal rings anteriorly, and slip a bougie past your finger into the trachea and advance it about 20 cm or until resistance is met. Remove your finger and then feed a 6.0 ETT over the bougie and inflate the cuff. Remove the bougie.

SUMMARY

Tracheostomy tubes are commonly encountered in the ED for patients with chronic respiratory disease and prolonged mechanical ventilation. Emergency physicians should be adept at identifying and managing life-threatening complications associated with tracheostomies, namely tube obstruction and tube dislodgement or decannulation. It is critically important to have a solid understanding of tracheostomy anatomy and use a practiced algorithmic approach to the tracheostomy patient in respiratory distress.

AWAKE FIBEROPTIC INTUBATION
Introduction

Management of the critical airway is an essential skill for any emergency physician. The emergency physician must also be able to identify a patient with a potentially difficult airway for whom facemask ventilation will be problematic or tracheal intubation is difficult or impossible. Fiberoptic intubation is regarded as an essential skill when a patient's airway is determined to be difficult.

Indications

The flexible fiberoptic scope (FFS) is a useful tool to navigate the airway. Fiberoptic intubation can be performed either nasally, orally or via tracheostomy. Use of a Williams Airway provides better glottic views and decreases intubation time when orally intubating.[39] The FFS is particularly useful in very anterior airways or obstructing airway masses that preclude visualization of the vocal cords even despite video laryngoscopy. If cervical instability is a concern, intubation with an FFS can be performed with less extension of the cervical spine than with traditional laryngoscopy. Real-time visualization of the fiberoptic scope passing through the vocal cords into the trachea provides a high level of confidence that an endotracheal tube can be passed off the fiberoptic scope into the trachea, and then visually confirmed to be correctly placed.[40]

Complications

Complications of FFS are uncommon but include epistaxis (with the nasal approach), laryngotracheal trauma, laryngospasm, and aspiration. Hypoxemia and aspiration are the most common complications associated with awake fiberoptic intubation.[41]

Fiberoptic intubation has been reported to have a first attempt failure rate of about 50%. Attempts were ultimately successful and were facilitated by ETT maneuvers, notably tube retraction and 90° counterclockwise rotation to avoid hang-up of the ETT on the right arytenoid cartilage.[40,42]

If there are copious airway secretions or blood in the airway, visualization via the fiberoptic camera can be easily obscured, making this method of intubation even more difficult.[43] Time to intubation is generally prolonged with awake fiberoptic intubation. Joseph and colleagues[42] found that fiberoptic intubation took 8 min longer than direct or video laryngoscopy in the operating room with a total procedure time of 24 min. Other pre-procedural considerations are all pre-intubation considerations including patient cooperation, time for adequate topical anesthetization and procedural sedation, and operator proficiency with the fiberoptic scope.

Combination of techniques

In select cases, combination techniques can be used such as the use of a laryngoscope blade to displace the tongue to promote endoscope passage. Combined video laryngoscopy and fiberoptic bronchoscopy is an excellent way to improve visualization of the glottis when there is an airway mass. In addition, combined laryngeal mask airway (LMA) with fiberoptic intubation helps in displacing the tongue and epiglottis while providing a track to advance the fiberoptic scope straight up to the aperture of the glottic opening.[40] This LMA method is at risk of displacing the ETT when attempting to remove the LMA, and the use of an Aintree Intubation Catheter can help mitigate this risk.[44]

Sedation and analgesia

Adequate sedation is critically important to achieve a successful first-pass attempt for awake fiberoptic intubation. There are many ways to approach sedation and anesthesia in an awake fiberoptic intubation. Topical anesthesia should always be performed and typically starts with lidocaine (or similar anesthetic) to decrease sensitivity in the nasal and oropharynx. Topicalization of the nasal mucosa will anesthetize the V1 and V2 divisions of the trigeminal nerve as well as the tongue, oropharynx, and larynx via the V3 division of the trigeminal nerve, glossopharyngeal, and vagus nerves can be topically anesthetized by application of gauze-soaked lidocaine gel, gargled viscous lidocaine, or nebulized lidocaine.[40]

In certain cases, moderate sedation will be required. It is a delicate balance to administer adequate sedation for a patient to be comfortable and cooperative during fiberoptic intubation while avoiding airway compromise from oversedation. The ideal level of sedation should result in a balance of patient comfort, cooperation, amnesia, hemodynamic stability, blunted airway reflexes and maintain a patent airway with spontaneous ventilation.[45] Benzodiazepines combined with opioids for awake fiberoptic intubation have been shown to increase the frequency of hypoxemia and apnea.[46] However, superior results have been shown for combination sedation using dexmedetomidine infusion plus midazolam[47] or dexmedetomidine infusion plus ketamine.[45]

In the ED, regional anesthesia is not typically an option, but it is interesting to note that a combination of sedation with conscious sedation and regional anesthesia with bilateral superior laryngeal nerve block can help reduce the time for fiberoptic intubation to just 14 min.[48,49]

Procedure

Basic preparation for difficult airway management includes having an available standard and emergency airway adjuncts (eg, supraglottic airway, gum-elastic bougie, and so forth), informing the patient with a known or difficult airway, assigning individuals to provide assistance when a difficult airway is encountered, preoxygenation by facemask, and administration of supplemental oxygen through the procedure. Adequate intravenous access and 20 mL of 2% lidocaine, dexmedetomidine infusion, and 100 mg of ketamine prepared.

1. For an awake fiberoptic intubation, the patient should be informed and aware of the procedure and steps involved. Reassurance should be provided that safety and comfort will be optimized. This can greatly help with patient anxiety and cooperation for the procedure.
2. Inject glycopyrrolate 0.2 mg intravenously for rapid onset antisalivary effect just before topical anesthesia.
3. For nasal approach, anesthetize the nasal mucosa using lidocaine 2% gel or 5% ointment.
   a. Gently dilate the selected nasal passage with lubricated nasopharyngeal airways of increasing diameter before passing an ETT.
4. For oral approach, maintain nasal cannula oxygen via the nares.
   a. Use an atomizer to spray 5 mL of 2% lidocaine directly on the visible portions of the tongue. Ask the patient to keep the drug in their mouth as long as possible.
   b. After 2 min, blindly spray another 5 mL of 2% lidocaine onto the posterior portion of the tongue and oropharynx.
   c. After 2 min, place a Williams Airway in the mouth.
5. Initiate an infusion of dexmedetomidine for conscious sedation. Bolus 1 mcg/kg over 10 min, followed by continuous infusion 0.5 mg/kg/h.
6. Administer 15 mg of intravenous ketamine after the dexmedetomidine bolus. An additional 20 mg of IV ketamine may be administered as needed for appropriate sedation.

7. Prepare a syringe with 10 mL of 2% lidocaine for injecting through the working channel of the fiberoptic scope.
8. Insert the tip of the fiberoptic scope through the Williams Airway and advance until the glottic region is visualized. Spray 4 mL of 2% lidocaine around and into the glottic opening, and then fully withdraw the scope.
9. If the patient is not already coughing, instruct them to cough twice to further diffuse the lidocaine.[48]
10. After 2 min, preload a lubricated ETT onto the fiberoptic bronchoscope. Be sure that the size of your ETT is appropriate for the size of the Williams Airway.
11. Reinsert the fiberoptic scope, now with ETT loaded, through the Williams Airway and introduce it through the vocal cords and visualize the trachea.
12. Advance the ETT over the fiberoptic scope into the trachea and confirm mid-tracheal positioning visually.
13. If there is difficulty advancing the ETT through the vocal cords, twist the ETT 90° counterclockwise rotation to avoid hang-up of the ETT on the right arytenoid cartilage.
14. Withdraw the scope and confirm good endotracheal placement with capnography and bilateral auscultation.
15. Confirm placement with portable CXR.

CLINICS CARE POINTS

- Ultrasound is a sensitive modality for diagnosing pleural effusion, complex effusion, and pneumothorax.
- Ultrasound-guided thoracentesis increases success rate and decreases complication rate.
- Patient positioning is important when accessing the pleural space. Upright position is preferred for pleural effusion.
- Contrary to traditional teaching, in hemothorax, smaller bore chest tubes may be preferable compared with large-bore chest tubes.
- In an obstructed tracheostomy emergency, remove the inner cannula and apply oxygen to patient's face and tracheostomy site.
- In a dislodged or decannulated tracheostomy, apply oxygen first to the face and tracheostomy site, and then follow a practiced algorithmic approach to reposition or remove the malpositioned tracheostomy tube.
- Combination video laryngoscopy-assisted fiberoptic bronchoscopy is an excellent way to increase first-pass intubation success when there is an airway mass.

Respiratory pathologies such as pneumothorax, hemothorax, tracheostomy dislodgement, and the difficult airway are life-threatening conditions that will be encountered in the ED. Emergency physicians should be able to promptly recognize these emergent pulmonary conditions and skillfully execute life-saving procedures such as thoracentesis, small- and large-bore tube thoracostomy, tracheostomy manipulation, and fiberoptic intubation. A variety of approaches are possible for every circumstance. However, with deference to and assimilation of evidence and recommendations in the current literature, we presented here our algorithmic approaches to each of these procedures and scenarios.

SUMMARY

To address difficult airways in the ED, the emergency medicine physician must be a master of the fiberoptic intubation. When visualization of the vocal cords is impossible with direct or video laryngoscopy because of an extremely anterior airway or obstructing airway mass, FFS is the method to use. Even with cervical instability, FFS can be used to intubate with minimal neck extension. Although an essential skill, fiberoptic intubation is infrequently used in the ED and requires prior planning, practice, and preparation.

DISCLOSURE

None.

REFERENCES

1. Ayres J GF. Imaging of the pleura. Semin Respir Crit Care Med 2010;31(6): 674–88.
2. Froudarakis M. Diagnostic work-up of pleural effusions. Respiration 2008; 75(1):4–13.
3. Noppen MDW. Volume and cellular content of normal pleural fluid in humans examined by pleural lavage. Am J Respir Crit Care Med 2000;162:1023–6.
4. Broaddus VC LR. Pleural effusion. In: Broaddus VC MR, editor. Murray and Nadel's textbook of respiratory medicine. Philadelphia: Elsevier; 2016.
5. Brown SGA BEW. Conservative versus interventional treatment for spontaneous pneumothorax. N Engl J Med 2020;382:405–15.
6. Al Omari A, Al-ashqar R, Alabd alrhman R, et al. Assessment of the harms and potential benefits of tracheostomy in COVID-19 patients: Narrative review of outcomes and recommendations. Am J Otolaryngol 2021;42(4):102972.
7. Alkrinawi S CV. Pleural infection in children. Semin Respir Infect 1996;11:148–54.
8. Blok B. Thoracentesis. In: Roberts JR, editor. Roberts and hedges' clinical procedures in emergency medicine and acute care. 7th edition. Philadelphia: Elsevier; 2019. p. 181–95.
9. Sahn S, Heffner J. Spontaneous pneumothorax. N Engl J Med 2020;342(12): 868–74.
10. Broaddus V. Clearing the air — a conservative option for spontaneous pneumothorax. N Engl J Med 2020;382:469–70.
11. Azfar AH, Lippmann M, Mundathaje U, et al. Spontaneous hemothorax: a comprehensive review. Chest 2008;134(5):1056–65.
12. Weldon EWJ. Pleural disease in the emergency department. Emerg Med Clin North Am 2012;30:475–99.
13. Yoon EA. A need to reconsider guidelines on management of primary spontaneous pneumothorax? Int J Emerg Med 2017. https://doi.org/10.1186/s12245-017-0135-x.
14. Young D, Harrison D, Cuthbertson B, et al. Effect of early vs late tracheostomy placement on survival in pateint receiving mechanical ventilation: the TracMan randomized trial. JAMA 2013;309(20):2121–9.
15. Davies H, Davies R, Davies C, BTS Pleural Disease Guideline Group. Mangement of pleural infection in adults: british thoracic society pleural disease guideline 2010. BMJ 2010;65(2):ii41–53.
16. Rahman N, Maskell N, Davies C, et al. The relationship between chest tube size and clinical outcoe in pleural infection. Chest 2010;137(3):536–43.
17. Yu H. Management of pleural effusion, empyema, and lung abscess. Semin Intervent Radiol 2011;28(1):75–86.
18. Chaddha U. Use of fibrinolytics and deoxyribonuclease in adult patients with pleural empyema: a consensus statement. Lancet Respir Med 2021;9:1050–64.

19. Chao T, Harbison S, Braslow B, et al. Outcomes after tracheostomy in COVID-19 patients. Ann Surg 2020;272:181–6.
20. Chaaban EA. Hepatic hydrothorax: an updated review on a challenging disease. Lung 2019;197(4). https://doi.org/10.1007/s00408-019-00231-6.
21. Tirado A, Wu T, Noble V, et al. Ultrasound-guided procedures in the emergency department - diagnostic and therapeutic asset. Emerg Med Clin North Am 2013; 31:117–49.
22. Bartter T, Mayo P, Pratter M, et al. Lower risk and higher yield for thoracentesis when performed by experienced operators. Chest 1993;103(6):1873.
23. Bauman MH, et al. Management of spontaneous pneumothorax an american college of chest physicians delphi consensus statement. Chest 2001;119(2): 590–602. https://doi.org/10.1378/chest.119.2.590.
24. Elyah O, Chatterji S. A review of symptoms and complications of ultrasound assisted thoracentesis in the first specialist pleural clinic in Israel. Isr Med Assoc J 2020;22(12):775.
25. Grogan D, Irwin R, Channick R, et al. Complications associated with thoracentesis. a prospective, randomized study comparing three different methods. Arch Intern Med 1990;150(4):873.
26. Seneff M, Corwin R, Gold L, et al. Complication associated with thoracocentesis. Chest 1986;90(1):97.
27. Joseph J, Viney S, Beck P, et al. A prospective study of amylase-rich pleural effusions with special reference to amylase isoenzyme analysis. Chest 1992; 102(5):1455.
28. Falcon-Chevere JMJC. Critical trauma skills and procedures in the emergency department. Emerg Med Clin North Am 2013;31(1):291–334. Available at: http://dxdoi.org/10.1016/j.emc.2012.09.004.
29. Bauman Z, Kulvatunyou N, Joseph B, et al. Randomized clinical trial of 14-french (14f) pigtail catheters versus 28-32f chest tubes in the management of patients with traumatic hemothorax and hemopneumothorax. World J Surg 2021;45(3): 880–6.
30. Bauman Z, Kulvatunyou N, Joseph B, et al. A prospective study of 7-year experience using percutaneous 15-french pigtail catheters for traumatic hemothorax/hemopneumothorax at a level-1 trauma center: size still does not matter. World J Surg 2018;42(1):107–13.
31. Kulvatunyou N, Bauman Z, Zein Edine S, et al. The small (14 Fr) percutaneous catheter (P-CAT) versus large (28-32 Fr) open chest tube for traumatic hemothorax: A multicenter randomized clinical trial. J Trauma Acute Care Surg 2021; 91(5):809–13.
32. Tanizaki S, Maeda S, Sera M, et al. Small tube thoracostomy (20-22 Fr) in emergent management of chest trauma. Injury 2017;48(9):1884–7.
33. Hooper C, Welham S, Maskell N. Pleural procedures and patient safety: a national BTS audit of practice. Thorax 2015;70:189–91.
34. Kasmani R, Irani F, Okoli K, et al. Re-expansion pulmonary edema followin thoracentesis. CMAJ 2010;182(18):2000–2.
35. Bontempo L, Manning S. Tracheostomy emergencies. Emerg Med Clin North Am 2019;37:109–19.
36. Fernandez-Bussy S, Mahajan B, Folch E, et al. Tracheostomy tube placement: early and late complications. J Bronchol Intervent Pulmonol 2015;22:357–64.
37. McGrath B, Bates L, Atkinson D, et al. Multidisciplinary guidelines for the management of tracheostomy and laryngectomy airway emergencies. Anaesthesia 2012;67:1025–41.

38. Long B, Koyfman A. Resuscitating the tracheostomy patient in the. Am J Emerg Med 2016;34:1148–55.

39. Greenland K, Lam M, Irwin M. Comparison of the williams airway intubator and ovassapian fibreoptic intubating airway for fibreoptic orotracheal intubation. Anaesthesia 2004;59:173–6.

40. Collins S, Blank R. Fiberoptic intubation: an overview and update. Respir Care 2014;59(6):865–80.

41. Ovassapian A. Fiberoptic endoscopy and the difficult airway. 2nd edition. Philadelphia: Lippincott Williams & Wilkins; 1996.

42. Joseph T, Gal J, DeMaria S, et al. A retrospective study of success, failure, and time needed to perform awake intubation. Anesthesiology 2016;125:105–14.

43. Hawkins E, Moy H, Brice J. Critical airway skills and procedures. Emerg Med Clin North Am 2013;31(1):1–28.

44. Berkow L, Schwartz J, Kan K, et al. Use of the laryngeal mask airway-aintree intubating catheter-fiberoptic bronchoscope technique for difficult intubation. J Clin Anesth 2011;23:534–9.

45. Sinha S, Chaudhary L, Hayaran N, et al. A comparision of dexmedetomidine plus ketamine combination with dexmedetomidine alone for awake fibertopic nasotracheal intubation: a randomized controlled study. J Anaesthesiol Clin Pharmacol 2014;30(4):514–9.

46. Bailey P, Pace N, Ashburn M, et al. Frequent hypoxemia and apnea after sedation with midazolam and fentanyl. Anesthesiology 1990;73:826–30.

47. Bergese S, Bender S, McSweeney T, et al. A comparative study of dexmedetomidine with midazolam and midazolam alone for sedation during elective awake fiberoptic intubation. J Clin Anesth 2010;22:35–40.

48. Ma Y, Cao X, Zhang H, et al. Awake fiberoptic orotracheal intubation: a protocol feasibility study. J Int Med Res 2021;49:1–10.

49. Macduff e a. Management of spontaneous pneumothorax: british thoracic society pleural disease guideline 2010. Thorax 2010;65(2):ii18–31. https://doi.org/10.1136/thx.2010.136986. Available at:.

Noninvasive Mechanical Ventilation

Harman S. Gill, MD[a,b], Evie G. Marcolini, MD[c,d],*

KEYWORDS

- Noninvasive ventilation • Continuous positive airway pressure
- Bilevel positive airway pressure • High flow nasal canula • Hypoxemia

KEY POINTS

- The most important benefit of noninvasive ventilation is to avoid the complications of intubation, which include ventilator-associated pneumonia, sinusitis, ICU delirium and critical illness myopathy.
- Noninvasive ventilation has been shown to reduce intubation rate, ICU or hospital length of stay, and mortality compared with standard simple oxygen therapy, with early application showing better outcomes.
- When considering noninvasive ventilation, it is best to use this modality early, before the patient has become severely acidotic or mental status diminishes to the point of not being safe to apply.
- Acidosis does not preclude the use of noninvasive ventilation.
- Application of a noninvasive device should be accompanied by close monitoring by either the physician, respiratory therapist, or nurse for an adequate period of time to determine whether the patient will tolerate the device, and whether the patient will maintain adequate mental status for airway protection.

INTRODUCTION

Noninvasive ventilation (NIV) is a relatively new concept, first introduced in the 1980s in the critical care setting, and now commonly used in the emergency medicine setting for patients with exacerbation of chronic obstructive pulmonary disease (COPD), cardiogenic pulmonary edema (CPE), pulmonary infiltrates in immunocompromised patients, and most recently patients with coronavirus disease 2019 (COVID-19)

a Department of Emergency Medicine, Section of Pulmonary & Critical Care Medicine, Geisel School of Medicine at Dartmouth; b Department of Medicine, Section of Pulmonary & Critical Care Medicine, Geisel School of Medicine at Dartmouth; c Department of Emergency Medicine, Division of Neurocritical Care, Geisel School of Medicine at Dartmouth; d Department of Neurology, Division of Neurocritical Care, Geisel School of Medicine at Dartmouth
* Corresponding author. Department of Emergency Medicine, Dartmouth-Hitchcock Medical Center, 1 Medical Center Drive, Lebanon, NH 03766.
E-mail address: emarcolini@gmail.com

Emerg Med Clin N Am 40 (2022) 603–613
https://doi.org/10.1016/j.emc.2022.05.010
0733-8627/22/© 2022 Elsevier Inc. All rights reserved.

infection with associated hypoxemia and ventilator failure. One survey showed that noninvasive ventilation use for COPD alone increased by 400% from 1998 to 2008 and was associated with a 42% reduction in invasive mechanical ventilation.[1]

This article explains the physiologic basis and fundamentals behind the technology of continuous positive airway pressure (CPAP), bilevel positive airway pressure (BPAP) and high flow nasal canula (HFNC); explores some of the core literature behind their clinical applications; and compares HFNC with other noninvasive modalities for respiratory failure alongside clinical titration and weaning algorithms in the emergency department setting.

The most important benefit of NIV is to avoid the complications of intubation, which include ventilator-associated pneumonia, sinusitis, ICU delirium, and critical illness myopathy. Furthermore, this modality also makes it possible for a patient to communicate, take in nutrition by mouth, and avoid the risks of sedation. The ventilatory support can benefit a patient in respiratory distress by decreasing the work of breathing and increasing effective ventilation. In this way, arterial oxygenation improves, and hypercapnia and respiratory acidosis are cleared. Compared with endotracheal intubation, NIV has been shown to lower the risk of infections, decrease the use of antibiotics, shorten length of stay in the ICU, and lower morbidity and mortality.[2] It is fair to say that the recent pandemic of COVID-19 has only further brought the value of NIV to the forefront, as ventilators became a scarce resource in many inundated communities. Historically, noninvasive mechanical ventilation has included tools such as negative pressure ventilators, iron lungs, pneumobelts, and rocking beds.[3] Fortunately, there are now portable modalities that can be easily implemented in the emergency department for patients with acute respiratory failure. These modalities include CPAP, BiPAP, and HFNC.

WHEN TO USE NONINVASIVE VENTILATION

When considering NIV, it is best to use this modality early, before the patient has become severely acidotic or mental status diminishes to the point of not being safe to apply. The patient should have adequate mental status in order to protect the airway from secretions or emesis. If the NIV is applied early, this can help to avoid endotracheal intubation, especially in patients with COPD and or CPE. Acidosis does not preclude the use of NIV, but a patient with pH below 7.3 may require more intensive care, thus warranting ICU-level nursing.

There are few absolute contraindications to NIV, including respiratory arrest, inability to appropriately fit a mask, inability of the patient to protect the airway, or facial trauma. Relative contraindications should be considered such as the patient with severe acidosis, hypotension, upper gastrointestinal (GI) bleeding, restraints, copious secretions, or recent upper airway or GI surgery. Any patient who is a candidate for endotracheal intubation should be considered for noninvasive ventilation, as this may improve the patient's physiology and obviate the need for endotracheal intubation. Patients who have a do not resuscitate status, or do not intubate status may also be considered for NIV, as it has been shown to be effective in resolving respiratory failure in 50% of patients who would otherwise have refused intubation.[4,5] Of note, a more contemporary use of NIV has been its use as an adjunctive preoxygenation modality to conventional and routine supplemental oxygen delivery interfaces by improving alveolar recruitment and oxygenation.

TYPES OF NONINVASIVE VENTILATION

Technically speaking, CPAP does not provide inspiratory aid, so to be precise it is not a true form of ventilation. It is nevertheless included in the category of noninvasive mechanical ventilation by consensus.[6] The physiology of CPAP is to provide continuous positive pressure through a closed circuit that raises functional residual capacity. This pressure recruits alveoli in patients with atelectasis and prevents alveolar collapse while decreasing the work of breathing. CPAP is similar to positive and expiratory pressure (PEEP) in the intubated and ventilated patient, although it can be challenging to control fraction of inspired oxygen (Fio_2) without the help of a mixer or a true ventilator.

BiPAP works by delivering inspiratory supportive pressure during the patient's inspiratory phase, maintaining a constant positive airway pressure and maintaining a predetermined positive pressure during expiratory phase, which provides the same support as CPAP or PEEP. A driving pressure is created, which is the difference between the inspiratory positive airway pressure (IPAP) and the expiratory positive airway pressure (EPAP) that assists with ventilation and allows for improvement of oxygenation. Although CPAP is helpful to patients with hypoxemic respiratory failure, BiPAP can be helpful in both hypoxemic and hypercapnic states, thus making it useful in the patient with COPD exacerbation.

The interface for CPAP and BIPAP can be one of many forms (**Figs. 1** and **2**). These include a full-face mask that incorporates both nose and mouth, full face mask that covers the entire face, nasal mask, mouthpiece, nasal pillows, or even a helmet. The most effective interface is likely that which creates a closed circuit, encapsulating mouth and nose; however, this may create a feeling of claustrophobia for the patient or skin breakdown over time. The helmet, mouthpiece, and nasal pillows place less mechanical force on the sensitive skin of the face and nose, but may not be as effective in creating positive pressure. Yet while each modality has proposed benefits and implications for patient-device interface tolerance and there are individual studies justifying noninferiority of a particular platform, there are no large, high-fidelity trials showing the superiority of 1 device interface compared with others in either hypoxemic or hypercarbic respiratory failure.

There are some practical considerations in applying noninvasive ventilation modes. After determining that a patient is a candidate for noninvasive ventilation, application of the device should be accompanied by close monitoring by either the physician, respiratory therapist ,or nurse for an adequate period of time in which to determine whether the patient will tolerate the device, and whether the patient will maintain adequate mental status for airway protection. Common predictors of failure include pH <7.25, Apache II score greater than 29, or Glasgow Coma Scale (GCS) less than 11. Clinician involvement is key to making sure that settings are appropriate and safety is maintained. If secretions are copious enough or do not improve with application, there is a high risk of failure or of developing pneumonia.

When choosing settings to initiate CPAP or BiPAP, it is advisable to start low and titrate up, monitoring patient comfort and maintaining tidal volumes around 6 to 8 mL/kg or a minute ventilation of 12 L. A common starting point is to start with IPAP 8 to 10 cm H_2O, and EPAP 4 to 6 cm H_2O; however, these settings may not be adequate for a patient with acute severe hypercapnia, and pressures should be titrated up swiftly with close monitoring. If pressures are too high, the patient can have discomfort, or there may be air leakage. Still, CPAP or PEEP should be maintained greater than 4 cm H_2O to avoid rebreathing. For patients with hypoxemia, a goal oxygen saturation (SpO2) greater than 90% may be followed, and incremental changes in Fio_2 and EPAP may be affected to attain this target. For patients with hypercarbia or combined oxygenation and ventilation deficits, the clinical parameter to target is minute ventilation (ideally somewhere between 8 and 10 L/min, but this is patient-specific). Strict attention should be paid to mask leak and average inspired

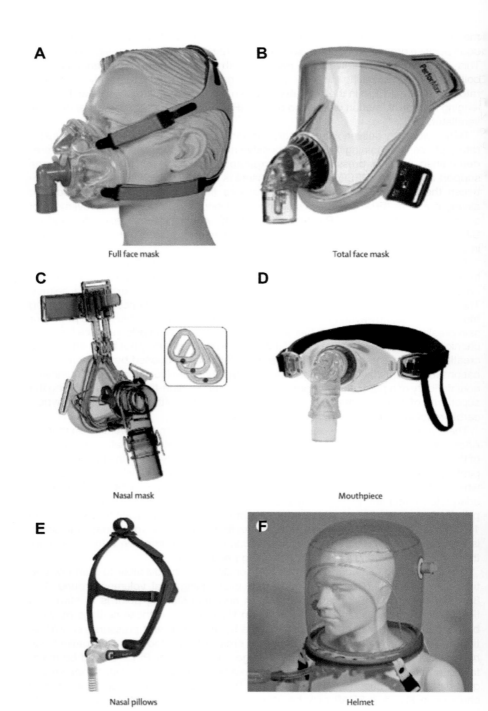

A Full face mask

B Total face mask

C Nasal mask

D Mouthpiece

E Nasal pillows

F Helmet

idal volumes so as to ensure that large and deleterious tidal volumes are not being delivered and volume trauma or barotrauma is not being caused.

CLINICAL APPLICATIONS

There are many clinical settings in which noninvasive ventilation can be applied. Noninvasive ventilation has been shown to reduce intubation rate, ICU or hospital length of stay, and mortality compared with standard simple oxygen therapy, with early application showing better outcomes.[7]

BiPAP should be considered in the setting of a COPD exacerbation when the $Paco_2$ is greater than 45 mm Hg, pH less than 7.35, and respiratory rate (RR) greater than 20 to 24 bpm. Conti and colleagues[8] showed that 48% of patients with COPD, failing standard medical treatment in the emergency department, avoided intubation, while having similar ICU mortality but lower readmissions in 1-year follow-up.

In the case of cardiogenic pulmonary edema (CPE), the literature is less compelling, because of small studies and exclusion of patients with cardiogenic shock or acute coronary syndrome. Multiple systematic reviews[9–13] have shown that noninvasive ventilation results in lower intubation and improved hospital mortality. These data showed similar benefits for CPAP or BiPAP, and overall showed that these modalities are not associated with an increase in myocardial infarction in the setting of CPE.

The patient with acute exacerbation of asthma experiences bronchoconstriction and limitation of expiratory airflow. This leads to breath stacking and hyperinflation, over which the patient must work to effectively breathe. This leads to increased work of breathing and a sense of dyspnea. Noninvasive ventilation can support this patient by providing a positive pressure, bringing air into the lungs, thus decreasing the pressure gradient and reducing the respiratory effort and work of breathing. This can help to avoid intubation while medical therapies address bronchoconstriction. Few prospective data exist to support the use of noninvasive ventilation for this patient population, although a recent retrospective review shows an increase in the use of noninvasive ventilation and no associated adverse events.[14]

Noninvasive ventilation has been investigated as an option for patients at end of life with respiratory failure and receiving comfort measures only but who wish to extend survival and/or provide comfort for a limited period of time.[15] Application of this mode of therapy must be preceded by a conversation with the patient and/or surrogated regarding goals of care and expectations for the therapy.

HIGH FLOW NASAL CANNULA

HFNC is a commonly used noninvasive modality for patients with respiratory failure in the emergency department. Although HFNC has primarily been studied in the literature and used clinically in the setting of hypoxemic respiratory failure, it is frequently used in other clinical domains also.

Circuit Basics

As described by Spoletini and colleagues, HFNC circuits are comprised of a water reservoir, an oxygen source/blender, a humidifier, a pressure release valve, and a

---

Fig. 1. Different types of interfaces. (*A*) Full face mask; (*B*) Total face mask; (*C*) Nasal mask; (*D*) Mouthpiece; (*E*) Nasal pillows; (*F*) Helmet. (*From* Nava S, Hill N. Non-invasive ventilation in acute respiratory failure. Lancet. 2009;374(9685):250-259. https://doi.org/10.1016/S0140-6736(09)60496-7.)

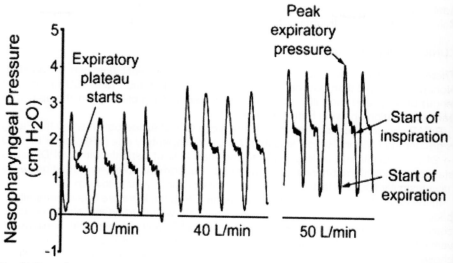

Fig. 2. Nasopharyngeal pressure generated by high-flow nasal cannula oxygen during the respiratory cycle at various flow rates in one patient postcardiac surgery. Each increase of 10 L/min raises mean airway pressure by 0.69 cm H_2O (closed) and 0.35 cm H_2O (open).

heated circuit in series.[16] As a result, these circuits allow accurate and reliable titration of 2 core physiologic variables in respiratory failure: air flow and fraction of inspired oxygen (Fio_2). Clinically, air flow addresses air hunger or respiratory fatigue, and accurate Fio_2 titration addresses hypoxemia. Low flow nasal canula (LFNC) systems or reservoir-based mask systems such as a nonrebreather or venturi masks are limited by flow rates and unreliable fractions of inspired oxygen that get delivered owing to issues with interface seal and entrainment of ambient air of lower Fio_2. In contrast, HFNC systems can have flow rates titrated from 20 L per minute (LPM) to 60 LPM with Fio_2 titrations in precise increments of 5% to 10%. This not only makes HFNC superior to LFNC or reservoir-based modalities, but also mimics the degree of Fio_2 and air flow support provided by invasive mechanical ventilators. Clinically, this has great advantages for the acute care clinician in the emergency department setting as treatment responders and nonresponders are predictable within an interval as short as 30 minutes.[17] Most HFNC systems should be started at 35 to 40 LPM at 100% Fio_2. A general rule is to titrate flow rate to respiratory rate by increments of 10 and target the lowest Fio_2 to achieve goal oxygen saturations. For instance, a patient breathing 40 bpm with oxygen saturation of 80% on a non-rebreather mask could be started at 40 LPM at 100% Fio_2. However, this aforementioned approach is not universal, as the impact of merely increasing flow rate can also improve oxygenation by reducing entrainment of ambient air with lower Fio_2, decrease work of breathing, and increase PEEP. If there is no improvement in oxygen saturation or tachypnea, early transition to invasive mechanical ventilation should be undertaken. Whereas, if the respiratory rate drops to 30 bpm and oxygen saturation is above goal, then the flow rate can also be deceased by an increment of 10 to 30 LPM and Fio_2 adjusted to goal oxygen saturation targets with frequent reassessments. Most patients can be safely weaned off HFNC to low flow systems when the flow rates are at or below 20 LPM and Fio_2 is at or below 50%.

Physiologic Rationale

Fundamentally, HFNC circuits derive their benefit by addressing 6 core clinical and physiologic concepts that have been rigorously studied in the literature: malleability; heat and humidification; moisture content of nasopharyngeal mucous, efficiency and the metabolic cost of breathing; reliable flow/Fio_2; and carbon dioxide (CO_2) washout.

As reported by Roca and colleagues, the wider diameter and longer length of the nasal prongs allow patients to comfortably receive supraphysiologic flow rates as high as 60 LPM.[18] In contrast, most patients on LFNC systems are remarkably intolerant of flow rates at or around 6 LPM. Part of this discomfort is owing to the narrow diameters and smaller nasal prongs, resulting in rapid insufflation but in large part also because of the lack of heat and humidification in these LFNC systems.

Work by Rittayamai and colleagues has shown that HFNC circuits can physiologically replicate the heat and humidification provided by the native nasopharynx even at flow rates as high as 60 LPM.[19] This work is further supported by Hasani and colleagues who showed a reduction in desiccation and epithelial injury by maintenance of this moisture content in the nasopharynx.[20] Furthermore, this moisture content allows improved ciliary clearance within the nasopharynx and maintenance of the inherent immunologic benefits of air filtration physiologically provided by the nares and cilia. Consequently, and as reported by Dysart and colleagues, HFNC reduces the metabolic work of breathing at such high flow rates.[21] Ultimately, these supraphysiologic flow rates allow reliable titration and delivery of Fio_2 because ambient air at 21% Fio_2 cannot be entrained into nasopharyngeal air that is being delivered at such high rates.[22] The robust rate of air flow combined with high fractions of inspired oxygen leads to a significant CO_2 washout also that then leads to a decrease in anatomic dead space in the tracheobronchial tree.[23]

Lastly, work from Parke and McGuinness has shown that each 10 L/min increase in air flow raises mean airway pressure in the hypopharynx by 0.69 cm H_2O in a fully closed circuit and 0.35 cm H_2O in a partially closed circuit.[24] In sum, HFNC circuits allow accurate titration of Fio_2 and air flow, maintain physiologic functions that are native to the nasopharynx and provide incremental increases in mean airway pressures in the hypopharynx.

Clinical Applications

One of the largest and earliest trials on the use of HFNC in acute hypoxemic respiratory failure was the work done by Frat and colleagues as part of the FLORALI study group and the REVA Network.[25] This study randomized an overall study population with acute hypoxemic respiratory failure to receive standard oxygen therapies (LFNC devices), conventional noninvasive ventilation (BIPAP/CPAP), or HFNC systems. Cumulative incidence of intubation in the overall population and a subgroup of patients with P_{AO_2}:Fio_2 $\leq$ 200 up to 28 days from enrollment and 90-day survival were studied in all 3 groups. Although the overall study population did show a lower incidence of intubation in the HFNC group, this outcome did not reach statistical significance. However, when a similar analysis was undertaken for the subgroup of patients with P_{AO_2}:Fio_2 (P:F) $\leq$ 200, HFNC use was associated with a statistically significant and lower incidence of intubation compared with LFNC and conventional noninvasive (NIV) modalities. Finally, HFNC also had a higher and statistically significant cumulative 90-day probability of survival when compared with LFNC and conventional NIV modalities. In sum, use of HFNC in patients with acute hypoxemic respiratory failure has been shown to decrease rates of eventual endotracheal intubation, especially in those with worse P:F ratios, and also to improve survival.

HFNC compared with other NIV modalities has been shown to be noninferior in preventing need for reintubation in patients with hypoxemia. In a study by Stephan and colleagues as part of the BiPOP study group, postoperative cardiothoracic surgical patients with hypoxemia were managed with either HFNC or BIPAP.[26] Treatment failure in this noninferiority trial was defined as need for reintubation, switching over to other study treatment or premature treatment discontinuation. Patients were monitored for 7 days after extubation, and there was no difference in the percent of patients without treatment failure between both arms of the study. P:F ratios increased in both groups but remained higher in the BIPAP group. Respiratory rates were higher with BIPAP and remained higher across the study timeframe. $Paco_2$, dyspnea and comfort scores were similar across both groups. In sum, HFNC is safe, effective and noninferior to traditional NIV modalities such as BIPAP in patients with type IV respiratory failure (postoperative atelectasis) and type I respiratory failure as shown by the FLORALI study.

Rittayamai and colleagues have also prospectively studied patients in an emergency department setting with acute dyspnea and hypoxemia.[19] They randomized patients to receive respiratory support for hypoxemia and dyspnea through conventional oxygen therapy or HFNC systems. Their primary outcomes were level of dyspnea, with secondary outcomes of comfort, changes in respiratory rate, adverse events, and rates of hospitalization. Patients receiving HFNC support for acute hypoxemia reported significant improvements in dyspnea and their overall comfort during their stay in the emergency department. Mean flow was 35 LPM in the HFNC arm and 6 LPM in the conventional therapy arm. No difference in hospital admission rates was observed. In sum, HFNC seems effective and robust in its evidence basis in improving dyspnea and alleviating respiratory fatigue in patients in the emergency department with acute hypoxia.

Further adjunctive use of HNFC both in and out of the emergency department with its associated support in the literature is summarized in **Table 1** by Spoletini and colleagues.[19,27–34]

Limitations, areas of controversy and further research

The COVID-19 pandemic has seen many patients in and out of the emergency department use HFNC systems during efforts of self-proning. Multiple studies have been published on the varied benefits of self-proning for patients with COVID-19, but the prescription of oxygen has been heterogenous in these studies, with support being provided by a mixture of LFNC, HFNC, and other NIV modalities. A head-to-head superiority or noninferiority trial assessing the ability of HFNC systems to prevent need for invasive mechanical ventilation or a mortality benefit has yet to be described in an emergency department setting.

A major area of controversy is the use of HFNC systems in patients with primarily hypercarbic respiratory failure. Much of the literature has studied combined hypoxic and hypercarbic respiratory failure. As reported earlier, there is physiologic evidence of a clear CO_2 washout and reduction of anatomic dead space fraction owing to a CO_2 sink created by the high flow rates inherent in HFNC circuits. But neither a consistent improvement in alveolar ventilation nor a reduction for need of mechanical ventilation and mortality have been reported like the classic literature supporting BIPAP/CPAP use in hypercarbic respiratory failure.

With regards to limitations, HFNC systems are more expensive than LFNC systems and need specialized monitoring and titration by trained professionals. These issues of cost and clinician training pose major barriers in its consistent use in the prehospital, austere, and resource-poor settings like developing countries. Furthermore, HFNC is

Table 1
Potential clinical applications of high-flow nasal oxygen

Application	Benefits
Procedures	Enhanced oxygenation during endoscopy[27]
Hypoxemic respiratory failure	
Acute respiratory distress syndrome	Mild and early[28]
Pneumonia	Enhanced oxygenation[18,17]
Idiopathic pulmonary fibrosis	Lower respiratory rate[29]
Cariogenic pulmonary fibrosis	Enhanced oxygenation Reduced dyspnea[28]
Postoperatively	
Cardiothoracic and vascular	Improved thoracoabdominal synchrony[35]
Cardiac surgery	Increased end-expiratory lung volume[19] Less escalation of therapy[21]
Postextubation	Improved oxygenation and ventilation[32] Enhanced comfort[33,19] Less displacement of interface[32] Less escalation of therapy to noninvasive ventilation or intubation[32]
Do-not-intubate patients	Improved oxygenation and respiratory mechanics[34]

From Spoletini G, Alotaibi M, Blasi F, Hill NS. Heated Humidified High-Flow Nasal Oxygen in Adults: Mechanisms of Action and Clinical Implications. Chest. 2015 Jul;148(1):253-261.

known to be more aerosolizingthan LFNC systems and requires the added precautions to maintain health care worker safety during pandemics such as COVID-19.

In summary, the noninvasive ventilatory modalities of CPAP, BiPAP, and HFNC are all beneficial in forestalling endotracheal intubation in the patient with respiratory distress. Understanding the physiologic basis and evidence-based applications for each will help optimize care with minimal invasiveness.

CLINICS CARE POINTS

- HFNC is a device that allows accurate titration of flow (5 L/min to 60 L/min) and Fio_2 (30% to 100%).
- Titrate flow incrementally by 10 L/min every 30 seconds to meet patients air hunger and respiratory rate.
- Start Fio_2 at 100%. If oxygenation targets are met, then titrate Fio_2 down by 5% every 30 seconds to meet goal oxygen saturations.
- When Fio_2 is at or below 35% and flow below 30 L/min, consider transition to low flow nasal cannula.
- If targets of oxygenation and reduction of work of breathing is not achieved with 30 minutes of starting therapy, then consider alternative noninvasive or invasive modalities for respiratory support.

DISCLOSURE

The authors have nothing to disclose.

REFERENCES

1. Mas A, Masip J. Noninvasive ventilation in acute respiratory failure. Int J Chron Obstruct Pulmon Dis 2014;9:837–52.
2. Girou E, Schortgen F, Delclaux C, et al. Association of noninvasive ventilation with nosocomial infections and survival in critically ill patients. JAMA 2000;284: 2361–7.
3. Ambrosino N, Vagheggini G. Noninvasive positive pressure ventilation in the acute care setting: where are we? Eur Respir J 2008;31(4):874–86.
4. Levy M, Tanios MA, Nelson D, et al. Outcomes of patients with do-not-intubate orders treated with noninvasive ventilation. Crit Care Med 2004;32:2002–7.
5. Schettino G, Altobelli N, Kacmarek RM. Noninvasive positive pressure ventilation reverses acute respiratory failure in selected "do-not-intubate" patients. Crit Care Med 2005;33:1976–82.
6. International Consensus Conference in Intensive Care Medicine: noninvasive positive pressure ventilation in acute respiratory failure. Am J Respir Crit Care Med 2001;163:283–91.
7. Lightowler JV, Wedzicha JA, Elliott MW, et al. Noninvasive positive pressure ventilation to treat respiratory failure resulting from exacerbations of chronic obstructive pulmonary disease: Cochrane systematic review and meta-analysis. BMJ 2003;326:185–9.
8. Conti G, Antonelli M, Navalesi P, et al. Noninvasive vs. conventional mechanical ventilation in patients with chronic obstructive pulmonary disease after failure of medical treatment in the ward: a randomized trial. Intensive Care Med 2002;28: 1701–7.
9. Potts JM. Noninvasive positive pressure ventilation: effect on mortality in acute cardiogenic pulmonary edema: a pragmatic meta-analysis. Pol Arch Med Wewn 2009;119:349–53.
10. Weng CL, Zhao YT, Liu QH, et al. Meta-analysis: noninvasive ventilation in acute cardiogenic pulmonary edema. Ann Intern Med 2010;152:590–600.
11. Mariani J, Macchia A, Belziti C, et al. Noninvasive ventilation in acute cardiogenic pulmonary edema: a meta-analysis of randomized controlled trials. J Card Fail 2011;17:850–9.
12. Vital FM, Ladeira MT, Atallah AN. Non-invasive positive pressure ventilation (CPAP or bilevel NPPV) for cardiogenic pulmonary oedema. Cochrane Database Syst Rev 2013;5:CD005351.
13. Cabrini L, Landoni G, Oriani A, et al. Noninvasive ventilation and survival in acute care settings: a comprehensive systematic review and metaanalysis of randomized controlled trials. Crit Care Med 2015;43:880–8.
14. Manglani R, Landaeta M, Maldonado M, et al. The use of non- invasive ventilation in asthma exacerbation - a two year retrospective analysis of outcomes. J Community Hosp Intern Med Perspec 2021;11(5):727–32.
15. Curtis JR, Cook DJ, Sinuff T, et al. Noninvasive positive pressure ventilation in critical and palliative care settings: understanding the goals of therapy. Crit Care Med 2007;35(3):932–9.
16. Spoletini G, Alotaibi M, Blasi F, et al. Heated Humidified High-Flow Nasal Oxygen in Adults: Mechanisms of Action and Clinical Implications. Chest 2015;148(1): 253–61.
17. Sztrymf B, Messika J, Mayot T, et al. Impact of high-flow nasal cannula oxygen therapy on intensive care unit patients with acute respiratory failure: a prospective observational study. J Crit Care 2012;27(3):e9–13.

18. Roca O, Riera J, Torres F, et al. High-flow oxygen therapy in acute respiratory failure. Respir Care 2010;55(4):408–13.
19. Rittayamai N, Tscheikuna J, Rujiwit P. High-flow nasal oxygen versus conventional oxygen therapy after endotracheal extubation: a randomized crossover physiologic study. Respir Care 2014;59(4):485–90.
20. Hasani A, Chapman TH, McCool D, et al. Domiciliary humidification improves lung mucociliary clearance in patients with bronchiectasis. Chron Respir Dis 2008;5(2):81–6.
21. Dysart K, Miller TL, Wolfson MR, et al. Research in high flow therapy: mechanisms of action. Respir Med 2009;103(10):1400–5.
22. Ritchie JE, Williams AB, Gerard C, et al. Evaluation of a humidified nasal high-flow oxygen system, using oxygraphy, capnography and measurement of upper airway pressures. Anaesth Intensive Care 2011;39(6):1103–10.
23. Sztrymf B, Messika J, Bertrand F, et al. Beneficial effects of humidified high flow nasal oxygen in critical care patients: a prospective pilot study. Intensive Care Med 2011;37(11):1780–6.
24. Parke RL, McGuinness SP. Pressures delivered by nasal high flow oxygen during all phases of the respiratory cycle. Respir Care 2013;58(10):1621–4.
25. Frat JP, Thille AW, Mercat A, et al, FLORALI Study Group; REVA Network. High-flow oxygen through nasal cannula in acute hypoxemic respiratory failure. N Engl J Med 2015;372(23):2185–96.
26. Stéphan F, Barrucand B, Petit P, et al, BiPOP Study Group. High-flow nasal oxygen vs noninvasive positive airway pressure in hypoxemic patients after cardiothoracic surgery: a randomized clinical trial. JAMA 2015;313(23):2331–9.
27. Lomas C, Roca O, Alvarez A, et al. Fibroscopy in patients with hypoxemic respiratory insufficiency: utility of the high-flow nasal cannula. Respir Med CME 2009; 2(3):121–4.
28. Frat J-P, Brugiere B, Ragot S, et al. Sequential application of oxygen therapy via high-flow nasal cannula and noninvasive ventilation in acute respiratory failure: an observational pilot study. Respir Care 2015;60(2):170–8.
29. Bräunlich J, Beyer D, Mai D, et al. Effects of nasal high flow on ventilation in volunteers, COPD and idiopathic pulmonary fibrosis patients. Respiration 2012; 85(4):319–25.
30. Corley A, Caruana LR, Barnett AG, et al. Oxygen delivery through high-flow nasal cannulae increase end-expiratory lung volume and reduce respiratory rate in post-cardiac surgical patients. Br J Anaesth 2011;107(6):998–1004.
31. Parke R, McGuinness S, Dixon R, et al. Open-label, phase II study of routine high-flow nasal oxygen therapy in cardiac surgical patients. Br J Anaesth 2013;111(6): 925–31.
32. Itagaki T, Okuda N, Tsunano Y, et al. Effect of high-flow nasal cannula on thoraco-abdominal synchrony in adult critically ill patients. Respir Care 2014;59(1):70–4.
33. Tiruvoipati R, Lewis D, Haji K, et al. High-flow nasal oxygen vs high-flow face mask: a randomized crossover trial in extubated patients. J Crit Care 2010; 25(3):463–8.
34. Epstein AS, Hartridge-Lambert SK, Ramaker JS, et al. Humidified high-flow nasal oxygen utilization in patients with cancer at Memorial Sloan-Kettering Cancer Center. J Palliat Med 2011;14(7):835–9.
35. Parke RL, McGuinness SP, Eccleston ML. A preliminary randomized controlled trial to assess effectiveness of nasal high-flow oxygen in intensive care patients. Respir Care 2011;56(3):265–70.

The Physiologically Difficult Intubation

Kenneth Butler, DO, Michael Winters, MD, MBA*

KEYWORDS

- Peri-intubation cardiac arrest • Peri-intubation cardiovascular collapse
- Preintubation hypoxemia • Preintubation hypotension • Shock index
- Intubation checklist

KEY POINTS

- The emergency physician should correct hypoxemia and provide adequate preoxygenation to critically ill emergency department (ED) patients before intubation.
- Consider initiation of a vasopressor infusion during rapid sequence intubation of the patient at high risk for cardiovascular collapse.
- Proper room setup and patient position are essential for successful intubation of the critically ill ED patient.
- Rapid sequence intubation medications should be selected and dosed accordingly in the critically ill ED patient.
- Consider smaller intravenous fluid boluses, early initiation of vasopressor medications, and pulmonary vasodilators when preparing to intubate the patient with pulmonary hypertension.

INTRODUCTION

More than 1.5 million critically ill patients are intubated each year in the United States.[1–3] Endotracheal intubation is a common procedure performed in the resuscitation and management of critically ill emergency department (ED) patients. Importantly, these patients often have anatomic and/or physiologic derangements that increase the risk of adverse outcomes, such as peri-intubation cardiovascular collapse and cardiac arrest. Risk factors for peri-intubation cardiovascular collapse and cardiac arrest in critically ill adult and pediatric patients include hypoxemia before intubation, hypotension before intubation, an elevated preintubation shock index, the absence of preoxygenation, and the need for emergent intubation.[4–6] In a recent multicenter study of more than 3600 critically ill patients who underwent tracheal intubation, more than 45%

Department of Emergency Medicine, University of Maryland School of Medicine, 110 South Paca Street, 6th Floor, Suite 200, Baltimore, MD 21201, USA
* Corresponding author.
E-mail address: mwinters@som.umaryland.edu

Emerg Med Clin N Am 40 (2022) 615–627
https://doi.org/10.1016/j.emc.2022.05.011
0733-8627/22/© 2022 Elsevier Inc. All rights reserved.

experienced at least one major adverse peri-intubation event.[7] In order to prevent adverse events that may result in poor patient outcomes, it is imperative that the emergency physician (EP) rapidly identify and appropriately resuscitate patients who are considered a "physiologically difficult intubation." The following chapter discusses crucial components of the evaluation and resuscitation of critically ill patients with anatomic and physiologic derangements who require ED intubation.

Anatomic Derangements

Predictors of the difficult airway

Assessment of the ED patient for anatomic abnormalities that predict a difficult intubation is standard practice in emergency medicine. Several bedside tests and measurements are commonly used to predict either a difficult airway or difficulty with bag-valve-mask (BVM) ventilation. Common tests and measurements include the Mallampati score, Wilson risk score, thyromental distance, sternomental distance, mouth opening, the upper lip bite test, neck mobility, and neck circumference. Although these assessments are expected to have high sensitivity in the identification of a potential difficult airway, their clinical utility remains unclear. A recent prospective cohort study of more than 2800 patients demonstrated that approximately 17% of airway-related adverse events were unanticipated and not predicted by common bedside airway assessments.[8] In another cohort study of more than 88,000 patients, almost 3,400 patients had a difficult tracheal intubation.[9] Of patients with a difficult intubation, more than 90% were unanticipated.[9] These findings imply that common bedside tests and measurements used to predict an anatomically difficult airway perform poorly as screening tests. Unfortunately, no single test accurately predicts a difficult airway. Thus, the EP should approach every intubation in a critically ill ED patient as a potential difficult airway.

Physiologic Derangements

Hypoxemia

Acute hypoxemic respiratory failure is a primary reason for endotracheal intubation and initiation of mechanical ventilation in the critically ill ED patient. Notwithstanding, hypoxemia before intubation is one of the strongest predictors of intubation-related adverse events and peri-intubation cardiac arrest in both adults and children.[4,6] As such, it is important for the EP to correct hypoxemia with the administration of supplemental oxygen before intubation of the critically ill ED patient.

Preoxygenation is the administration of oxygen to a patient before intubation in order to extend the safe apnea time required for successful endotracheal tube insertion. A recent consensus statement from the Society for Airway Management recommends that all patients be maximally preoxygenated before intubation.[10] Preoxygenation increases the fraction of alveolar oxygen, increases arterial oxygen tension, and decreases the fraction of alveolar nitrogen. The efficiency of preoxygenation is reflected in the rate of decline in oxyhemoglobin desaturation during apnea.[11] Optimal preoxygenation extends the time to desaturation in chemically induced apnea and improves the likelihood of first-pass success. Common endpoints that indicate optimal preoxygenation include an end-tidal oxygen concentration of 90% and an end-tidal nitrogen concentration of 5%.[10,12,13] In a healthy patient who has been preoxygenated for approximately 3 to 5 minutes or 8 vital capacity breaths, the average time to desaturation to levels less than 90% is approximately 8 minutes.[14] In contrast, critically ill patients more rapidly desaturate and have an increased risk for arrhythmias and hemodynamic instability during the intubation attempt.

Preoxygenation can be performed with several modalities that include a nonrebreather mask (NRM), high-flow nasal cannula (HFNC), BVM, or noninvasive positive pressure ventilation (NIPPV). The EP should select the best modality necessary to maintain adequate oxygen saturation. Often, an NRM is selected for preoxygenation. It is important to set the NRM at flush rate, rather than the traditional setting of 15 LPM.[10] Unfortunately, many NRMs do not maintain a tight seal against the patient's face. The lack of a tight seal allows room air to be pulled into the NRM and, thereby, decreases the fraction of inspired oxygen that is delivered to the patient. When using an NRM for preoxygenation, the authors of this chapter recommend the added use of a conventional nasal cannula set at 15 LPM, a practice referred to as apneic oxygenation. This conventional nasal cannula remains in place during the intubation procedure. Apneic oxygenation has been shown to improve safe apnea time in critically ill patients in various clinical settings.[10,15–17] Importantly, apneic oxygenation alone will not prevent adverse events if preoxygenation has been insufficient.[10] HFNC can be used for preoxygenation in patients who fail to achieve adequate saturation targets with an NRM set at flush rate. HFNCs are commercial devices that deliver heated and humidified oxygen at high flow rates (ie, 40–70 LPM) and is often well tolerated by patients compared with NIPPV. Whether HFNC devices provide a small amount of positive airway pressure remains controversial. Similar to a conventional nasal cannula, HFNCs can be left in place during laryngoscopy, as they do not obscure the laryngoscopic view. A BVM with a positive end-expiratory pressure (PEEP) valve or NIPPV should be used for preoxygenation in patients unable to achieve target oxygen saturation goals with either an NRM at flush rate or a HFNC device. In a recent randomized trial that involved critically ill adults who underwent tracheal intubation, patients who received BVM ventilation during the interval between induction and laryngoscopy had higher oxygen saturations and lower rates of severe hypoxemia than those receiving no BVM ventilation.[18] If a BVM is used for preoxygenation and to assist ventilation during induction, the PEEP valve should be set to 5 to 10 cm H2O.[10] In addition, if BVM ventilation is needed during induction, the authors recommend a 2-person technique to optimize ventilation. If NIPPV is used, either continuous positive airway pressure or bilevel positive airway pressure can be applied.

Regardless of the modality chosen, critically ill patients should be preoxygenated in the upright position.[10] Preoxygenation in an upright position has been shown to improve functional residual capacity and increase the safe apnea time.[10,19]

Hypotension

Similar to preintubation hypoxemia, hypotension before intubation is another strong predictor of peri-intubation cardiovascular collapse and cardiac arrest.[4,6] Although thresholds vary between studies, general hemodynamic thresholds for hypotension include a systolic blood pressure (SBP) less than 90 mm Hg or a mean arterial blood pressure (MAP) less than 65 mm Hg. In addition, an elevated shock index (SI) has also been shown to predict peri-intubation cardiovascular collapse.[20] The SI is calculated as the heart rate divided by the SBP, with the normal range between 0.5 and 0.7. Shock index values greater than 0.8 are associated with postintubation hypotension (PIH), whereas SI values greater than 0.9 are associated with postintubation cardiac arrest.[10,20–23]

Even in the absence of overt preintubation hypotension, critically ill ED patients are at significant risk of PIH. In fact, PIH occurs in up to 25% of ED intubations and is associated with increased mortality and increased lengths of stay in the intensive care unit.[22] The causes of PIH are multifactorial and can include abrupt loss of adrenergic tone due to sedative and paralytic medications used during rapid sequence intubation

(RSI), an abrupt increase in intrathoracic pressure due to the initiation of positive pressure ventilation, preexisting intravascular volume depletion, and severe acidosis. It is paramount for the EP to identify and resuscitate hypotensive patients at risk of peri-intubation cardiovascular collapse before intubation.

Intravenous fluids (IVFs) are commonly administered to hypotensive ED patients, or those at risk of PIH, to prevent cardiovascular collapse during RSI. Despite common practice, there remains scant evidence to demonstrate that IVFs prevent PIH and peri-intubation cardiovascular collapse. In a recent multicenter randomized trial of adult patients undergoing tracheal intubation, Janz and colleagues demonstrated no change in the composite outcome of hypotension, initiation of vasopressors, cardiac arrest, or death in patients who received IVFs during intubation compared with those who did not receive IVFs.[24] Admittedly, the trial was stopped early, and patients randomized to IVFs were only given 500 mL of crystalloid solution. Although the administration of IVFs to critically ill patients during RSI is likely to remain a common practice, it is important for the EP to recognize that IVFs alone may not prevent peri-intubation cardiovascular collapse. For the hypotensive patient who requires intubation in the setting of hemorrhagic shock, blood product transfusion should be considered in lieu of IVF administration.

For critically ill ED patients who require intubation and are at high risk for peri-intubation cardiovascular collapse, the authors recommend preparation of a vasopressor infusion. Over the past several years in emergency medicine, the administration of "push-dose pressors" (PDPs) or "bolus-dose pressors" has become common for the treatment of PIH and postarrest hypotension. In these circumstances, either epinephrine or phenylephrine is intermittently administered to improve SBP or MAP. Although PDPs are commonly used in the ED, the limited amount of literature on their use in the critically ill ED patient demonstrates significant adverse event and medication error rates.[25,26] It is for this reason that the authors feel a safer and more consistent method to administer vasopressor medications is through an infusion rather than a PDP. Consistent with most critical illness states, norepinephrine is recommended as the first-line vasopressor agent for infusion in patients with preintubation hypotension.[10] In a recent prospective cohort study, Smischney and colleagues found that a systolic blood pressure less than 130 mm Hg and a MAP less than 65 mm Hg were among several variables independently associated with PIH.[27] Thus, the authors recommend targeting an MAP of at least 65 mm Hg or an SBP of at least 130 mm Hg when titrating a vasopressor infusion before RSI.

Importantly, a central venous catheter is not required for the initiation of vasopressor medications. Several recent studies have demonstrated the safety of vasopressor administration through a properly placed peripheral intravenous catheter.[28–30] The incidence of extravasation and injury is lowest when peripheral catheters are placed at or above the antecubital fossa and are 20 gauge or larger in size.

Severe acidosis

Critically ill ED patients often have significant acid-base disturbances that markedly increase the risk for peri-intubation adverse events. In patients with a severe metabolic acidosis, respiratory compensation with hyperventilation may already be maximized.[10,31] Any reduction in respiratory rate during RSI will increase carbon dioxide concentration, further decrease arterial pH, and may result in a peri-intubation cardiac arrest.[10,29] In these very high-risk patients, it may be possible to avoid intubation with the use of HFNC or NIPPV; however, these modalities must be used with great caution especially if the patient exhibits altered mental status. If intubation cannot be avoided in patients with a severe metabolic acidosis, the Society for Airway Management recommends preoxygenation with NIPPV to estimate the patient's minute ventilation needs.[10] For patients with high minute ventilation needs, the EP should consider an awake intubation rather than RSI (see later under Special Considerations).[10,31] If an awake intubation cannot be performed or is unsuccessful and RSI is needed, the EP should consider a short-acting paralytic medication so that spontaneous breathing can be resumed with mechanical ventilation.[10] The routine administration of sodium bicarbonate to severely acidotic patients that require intubation has not been shown to prevent adverse outcomes and is not currently recommended.[10]

Preparation and Intubation

The intubation checklist

Intubation of the critically ill ED patient is a high-risk, high-stress procedure that can result in aspiration, critical hypoxia, cardiovascular collapse, permanent neurologic damage, and death if not properly performed. The risk of adverse events is reported to be 30 times greater when intubation is performed in the ED compared with more controlled environments, such as the operating room.[32] Factors that contribute to adverse events and poor outcomes include the failure to resuscitate patients before intubation, improper patient positioning, incorrect doses of RSI medications, failure to assemble the correct equipment needed to successfully intubate the patient, and failure to develop and verbalize a backup plan in the event of a failed attempt.[33] Furthermore, acutely stressful situations can impair vital cognitive functions, such as situational awareness, decision-making, problem solving, and memory recall. It is for these reasons that an intubation checklist has been suggested by many to provide a structured approach to the procedure and allow cognitive offload in this high-risk, high-stress circumstance. Similar to a "time out" that is taken before a surgical procedure, the intubation checklist provides the opportunity to ensure that all team members have a shared mental model of the intubation and the steps to be taken in the event of first-attempt failure. At present, the literature on intubation checklists in the ED is scant and the topic remains controversial. Notwithstanding, the authors of this chapter find value in the intubation checklist and recommend its use.

Importantly, an intubation checklist should be concise, easy to read, and contain the appropriate information so that actions can be performed correctly during the intubation attempt. In addition, checklists should be rapidly accessible, easily visualized, and easy to complete in the electronic health record. Each institution should develop its own checklist based on the patient population and institutional resources. A sample intubation checklist from the authors' institution is provided in **Fig. 1**.

The setup

Preparation is an essential component in the successful intubation of the critically ill patient with a physiologically difficult airway. Appropriate preparation of the patient and the room includes proper patient monitoring, patient positioning, suction, oxygen, and airway equipment. All critically ill patients who require intubation should be placed on continuous cardiac monitor, continuous pulse oximetry, and capnography. If an arterial line is not in place, frequent noninvasive blood pressure measurements should occur throughout the induction, laryngoscopy, and postintubation periods. It is important to place the noninvasive blood pressure cuff on the upper extremity opposite to the peripheral intravenous line used to administer RSI medications. To improve the airway axis and decrease the risk of aspiration, the head of the bed should be elevated such that the patient's external auditory canal is in line with the sternal notch. In addition to proper patient position, the authors recommend 2 suction setups, especially in critically ill patients with upper gastrointestinal hemorrhage or massive hemoptysis. As

ED INTUBATION CHECKLIST		
Patient Name:	Wt:	Allergies:

PEOPLE (Limit Non-Essential Staff inside room: 3 for intubation)

☐ Airway Operator   ☐ RN   ☐ RT

☐ MD & RNs outside the room (supplies, communication, documentation)

PREPARATION

☐ Adequate PPE (PAPR, Gown, Gloves x2, Shoe covers [optional])
☐ Appropriate room (negative pressure room for isolated airway)
☐ Audio communication set up

EQUIPMENT

GLIDESCOPE	AIRWAY BOX	ROOM SET-UP	COVID INTUBATION BAG

☐ Glidescope*
 ☐ S3 or S4 blade
 ☐ Stylet
	☐ 7.0 and 8.0 ETT
	 ☐ Bougie
	 ☐ Oral airway
	    +/- Nasal trumpet
	 ☐ Colorimetric
	    capnometer
		☐ Ambu Bag with PEEP Valve
		    & Viral Filter
		 ☐ Suction canister & tubing
		 ☐ Yankauer
		 ☐ ETCO2 "brick" + cord
			▪ Viral filter
			 ▪ Plastic drape
			 ▪ 10cc syringe (x2)
			 ▪ Adjustable thumb clamp
			 ▪ NGT/OGT
			 ▪ Piston Syringe
			 ▪ Tape Measure
			 ▪ $ETCO_2$ sampling line

PATIENT

☐ Adequate IV or IO access
☐ BP support (IVF, norepinephrine gtt) at bedside

PHARMACOLOGY

RSI MEDICATIONS	POST-INTUBATION ANALGOSEDATION	REMINDERS
Sedative (Select One) ☐ Etomidate 0.3 mg/kg ☐ Propofol 1-2 mg/kg ☐ Ketamine 1-2 mg/kg Paralytic (Select One) ☐ Rocuronium 1.2-1.5 mg/kg ☐ Vecuronium 0.3-0.6 mg/kg ☐ Succinylcholine 1-1.5mg/kg	Sedation ☐ Propofol gtt OR Midazolam gtt Analgesia • Scheduled IV/PO Opiates + PRN IV Opiates • Utilize continuous infusion only if necessary	Take EVERYTHING that will be needed (including post-intubation meds and procedure items) into the room BEFORE intubation. The door should be closed for ~ 30 min after intubation due to potential aerosols.

Fig. 1. Adapted from the RSI Checklist, University of Maryland Medical Center, Adult Emergency Department. * indicates the the video laryngoscope product used at the University of Maryland Medical Center. It is the GlideScope manufactured by Verathon.

discussed, adequate preoxygenation is essential to decrease the risk of peri-intubation cardiovascular collapse and peri-intubation cardiac arrest. One of the most common errors that occurs in RSI is a disconnected oxygen source. The EP must ensure that oxygen is connected and properly flowing to the device used for preoxygenation.

The authors recommend that the following airway equipment be at the bedside for RSI in the critically ill patient with a physiologically difficult airway: 2 endotracheal tubes configured with a malleable stylet that is straight-to-cuff with a 25- to 30-degree angle at the cuff, a video or direct laryngoscope, a Macintosh 4 laryngoscope blade, and a gum elastic bougie and supraglottic airway device should initial attempts at intubation be unsuccessful. As with all intubations in the ED, surgical airway equipment should be at the bedside in the event of failed endotracheal intubation and when confronted with a "can't intubate, can't ventilate" scenario.

Rapid sequence intubation medications

The selection and dose of sedative and paralytic medications for RSI of the ED patient with a physiologically difficult airway is paramount. The optimal sedative medication for RSI should have a rapid onset, short duration of action, minimal hemodynamic effect, minimal side-effect profile, and be rapidly reversible. Unfortunately, the ideal sedative medication for RSI of the ED patient does not exist. Each medication has advantages and disadvantages. The most common sedative medications used for RSI in the ED are listed in **Table 1**. In the critically ill ED patient with hypotension, the authors recommend a reduction in the dose of the sedative medication, as these medications can worsen hemodynamic status.

Similar to sedative medications, there is no ideal paralytic medication for RSI of every ED patient. Whether to routinely select a depolarizing paralytic medication (ie, succinylcholine) or a nondepolarizing paralytic medication (ie, rocuronium) remains controversial, depending on the clinical situation, and, often, is a matter of personal preference and experience. The most common paralytic medications used for RSI in the ED are listed in **Table 2**. The authors of this chapter prefer a nondepolarizing paralytic medication to ensure optimal conditions for intubation. In the event of a failed intubation, the use of a longer acting nondepolarizing medication provides for easier BVM ventilation, insertion of a supraglottic airway, or another attempt at intubation compared with a patient who may awaken after the use of a depolarizing agent for RSI. If rocuronium is selected as the paralytic agent in a critically ill ED patient with hypotension, a recent analysis of the National Emergency Airway Registry demonstrated a higher first-attempt success rate with doses greater than or equal to 1.4 mg/kg.[34]

Special Considerations

Awake intubation

An awake intubation is simply the insertion of the endotracheal tube while the patient continues to spontaneously breathe. The principal advantage to an awake intubation over RSI is that you do not take away the patient's airway reflexes and spontaneous respirations.[35] The ability of the patient to maintain both spontaneous ventilation and intrinsic airway tone may lead to more favorable patient safety conditions while the trachea is intubated.[36–38] The ideal candidate for an awake intubation is the noncrashing ED patient in whom the loss of airway reflexes during RSI can result in dire consequences, should intubation be unsuccessful. In general, the EP should consider an awake intubation in ED patients who have difficult airway features, progressive loss of airway anatomy over time, and in whom intubation is less urgent. Common conditions in which awake intubation is used include ED patients with severe metabolic acidosis, angioedema, nonangioedema airway obstruction, oropharyngeal infections, neck trauma, or those with altered oral or laryngeal anatomy. The primary disadvantages of an awake intubation are that it requires the full cooperation of the patient and management of their airway reflexes.

Awake intubation does not require any additional skills beyond standard intubation skills, the ability to manage a difficult airway, and the ability to perform a surgical airway, if needed. An awake intubation consists of a 3-part procedure: drying secretions, topical anesthesia, and sedation followed by intubation.

Table 1
Sedative medications

Medications	Dose	Onset	Duration	Advantages	Drawbacks
Etomidate	0.3 mg/kg	10–15 s	5–15 min	Minimal hemodynamic side effects; cerebral perfusion pressure well maintained	Myoclonus; pain at injection site; transient adrenal suppression
Ketamine	1.5 mg/kg (4 mg/kg IM)	60–90 s	10–20 min	Favorable hemodynamic profile; can be used in TBI as it maintains cerebral perfusion pressure; can be used in reactive airway disease	Has negative inotropic effect and may worsen hypotension in select patients; laryngospasm may be seen in awake intubations
Propofol	1.5 mg/kg	30–40 s	4–6 min	Can be used in reactive airway disease and in cases of status epilepticus	Myocardial depression; pain at injection site; reduces cerebral perfusion pressure

- Drying secretions: the effect of topical anesthesia is enhanced when applied to dry mucosa. To dry the mucosa, the authors recommend the administration of glycopyrrolate (0.2 mg intravenously [IV] or intramuscularly [IM]).[39] Atropine (0.5–1.0 mg IV or IM) can be used as an alternative if there are no concerns over its hemodynamic effects on the patient. After administration of the antisialagogue, the EP should use gauze pads to physically dry the tongue and oropharynx.
- Topical anesthesia: if time permits, the authors recommend administration of 4% liquid lidocaine delivered through a nebulizer at low flow rates (4–8 L per minute). This low flow rate will prevent the anesthetic from going too deep into the tracheobronchial tree.[40] During the nebulizer treatment, the EP should instruct the patient to extend the tongue in order to increase the delivery of the medication to the pharynx. After the administration of nebulized lidocaine, 4% liquid lidocaine is sprayed onto the tonsillar pillars with an atomizer device.[41,42] The EP can use gauze to hold the patient's tongue forward while atomizing lidocaine to the oropharynx. Finally, 2% viscous lidocaine can be placed on a tongue depressor and dripped down the patient's pharynx for additional anesthesia.
- Sedation: ketamine is an ideal sedative medication for awake intubation, as it preserves the patient's intrinsic airway reflexes and respiratory drive.[40] Ketamine should be administered at a lower, procedural sedation dose for an awake intubation (0.1–0.5 mg/kg IV or 3 mg/kg IM). In the authors' experience, 20 mg boluses of ketamine, titrated to effect, work well for awake intubation in cooperative patients. In uncooperative or agitated patients, higher doses of ketamine can be used (ie, 1.5 mg/kg), although it is important to recognize that apnea and/or laryngospasm are more likely with higher doses. Benzodiazepine medications can also be used for sedation in awake intubation when ketamine is not available.

Table 2
Paralytic medications

Medications	Dose	Onset	Duration	Advantages	Drawbacks
Succinylcholine	1.5 mg/kg (4 mg/kg IM)	45–60 s	6–10 min	Ideal if needing to extubate a patient following a procedure or if needed to assess the neurologic examination in an intubated patient	Contraindicated in hyperkalemia, malignant hyperthermia, neuromuscular disorders, or more than 5 d after a crush or burn injury; fasciculation; elevated intraocular pressure
Rocuronium	1.5 mg/kg	45–60 s	20–35 min	Widely used, given lack of adverse effects seen with succinylcholine	
Vecuronium	1.3 mg/kg	45–60 s	More than 35 min	High dose may provide an alternative means of achieving rapid-onset blockade; minimal cardiovascular effects	

Traumatic brain injury

Hypotension, hypoxia, and hypercarbia worsen outcome in patients with traumatic brain injury (TBI) and must be avoided. Failure to control the airway in ED patients with TBI who require intubation may lead to, or worsen, hypoxia and hypercapnia. In addition, injudicious use of medications during RSI, along with the application of positive pressure ventilation, can cause hypotension and result in harmful decreases in cerebral perfusion pressure. In contrast, inadequate sedation during laryngoscopy can precipitate hypertension and increase intracranial pressure, which may further worsen neurologic injury in these tenuous patients.

Given the potential perils of RSI in the patient with TBI, it is imperative to optimize conditions to ensure first-attempt success. Appropriate preoxygenation before intubation cannot be overemphasized for RSI of the ED patient with TBI. Although apneic oxygenation is beneficial, it will not rescue inadequate preoxygenation.[10] Importantly, the degree of obtundation in a patient with TBI does not correlate with the degree of an exaggerated sympathetic reflex that can occur with laryngoscopy. Although it has not been shown to consistently blunt the sympathetic reflex in patients with TBI, fentanyl can be considered. In regard to sedation, etomidate is preferred by many for RSI in patients with TBI due to its favorable hemodynamic profile. In fact, etomidate has been shown to decrease cerebral blood flow, decrease cerebral metabolic demand, and preserve cerebral perfusion pressure.[43] Importantly, etomidate does not have analgesic properties and will require an analgesic to be given early in the postintubation period. In recent years, ketamine has gained traction for use in patients with TBI and may be ideal in the setting of normal to low preintubation blood pressure.[44] In regard to paralytic medications, succinylcholine may increase intracranial pressure and also increase oxygen consumption due to fasciculations. In a comparative study of ED patients with severe brain injury, succinylcholine was associated with increased mortality when compared with rocuronium for those with a high Abbreviated Injury Scale score.[45] For these reasons, the authors of this chapter believe that rocuronium is the paralytic agent of choice in ED patients with TBI.

Pulmonary hypertension

Patients with acute or chronic pulmonary hypertension are at high risk for peri-intubation cardiovascular collapse and cardiac arrest during RSI. For an in-depth discussion on pulmonary hypertension, please see the accompanying chapter in this edition by Dr Sara Crager titled *Pulmonary Hypertension*. In essence, worsened hypoxemia or hypercapnia during RSI will increase pulmonary vasoconstriction and lead to an increase pulmonary vascular resistance and an increase in afterload to the compromised right ventricle (RV). In addition, the initiation of positive pressure ventilation will also increase RV afterload and further compromise RV output. These combined effects increase RV wall tension and RV oxygen consumption and result in RV failure, left ventricular failure, and, ultimately, cardiac arrest. In fact, intubation of the patient with pulmonary hypertension may be the most physiologically difficult airway the EP will encounter.

Before intubation of the patient with pulmonary hypertension, it is important to evaluate volume responsiveness of the RV.[10] Indiscriminate fluid administration to the patient with a dilated RV can further displace the intraventricular septum and impair left ventricular output. In patients with evidence of RV overload, diuresis may be indicated before RSI.[10] In addition, inhaled or intravenous pulmonary vasodilators can be considered in these patients to decrease RV afterload.[10] For volume responsive patients with pulmonary hypertension, the Society for Airway Management recommends smaller fluid boluses (ie, 250 mL) in contrast to large volume fluid administration.[10] Vasopressor medications (ie, norepinephrine) should be prepared and present in the room before initiation of RSI in patients with pulmonary hypertension. For patients with chronic pulmonary hypertension, current recommendations are to target a higher mean arterial blood pressure to ensure adequate coronary perfusion pressure during intubation.[10] Finally, hypoxemia and hypercapnia should be avoided during RSI, thereby emphasizing the need to appropriate and adequately preoxygenate the patient before RSI.

SUMMARY

Emergency physicians intubate critically ill patients almost daily. Intubation of the critically ill ED patient is a high-risk, high-stress situation, as many have physiologic derangements such as hypotension, hypoxemia, acidosis, and RV dysfunction that markedly increase the risk of peri-intubation cardiovascular collapse and cardiac arrest. In order to prevent disastrous peri-intubation outcomes, it is imperative for the EP to use the tips discussed in this article to improve the physiology of these patients before intubation. These tips include appropriate preoxygenation, correction of hypotension, patient position, setup of the room, proper selection and doses of RSI medications, and consideration of awake intubation in select patients.

CLINICS CARE POINTS

- When intubating the critically ill patient, correct hypoxemia and hypotension before administering RSI medications and performing laryngoscopy.
- Use a checklist when performing RSI in the critically ill ED patient to ensure proper setup.
- When performing an awake intubation in a patient with severe metabolic acidosis, ensure that an appropriate amount of topical anesthesia is administered.
- When intubating the patient with traumatic brain injury, avoid hypotension, hypoxia, and hypercarbia.

DISCLOSURE

The authors have nothing to disclose.

REFERENCES

1. Heideger T. Management of the difficult airway. N Engl J Med 2021;384:1836–47.
2. Pfunter A, Wier LM, Stocks C. Most frequent procedures performed in US hospitals, 2011: statistical brief #165. In: Agency for healthcare research and quality, editor. Healthcare cost and utilization project (HCUP) statistical briefs. Agency for Healthcare Research and Quality; 2013. p. 1–10.
3. Driver BE, Semler MW, Wesley H, et al. Effect of use of a bougie vs endotracheal tube with stylet on successful intubation on the first attempt among critically ill patients undergoing tracheal intubation. JAMA 2021;326(24):2488–97. Published online December 8, 2021.
4. De Jong A, Rolle A, Molinari N, et al. Cardiac arrest and mortality related to intubation procedure in critically ill adult patients: A multicenter study. Crit Care Med 2018;46:532–9.
5. April MD, Arana A, Reynolds JC, et al. Peri-intubation cardiac arrest in the emergency department: A National Emergency Airway Registry (NEAR) study. Resuscitation 2021;162:403–11.
6. Pokrajac N, Sbiroli E, Hollenbach KA, et al. Risk factors for peri-intubation cardiac arrest in a pediatric emergency department. Pediatr Emerg Care 2022;38: e126–31.
7. Russotto V, Myatra SN, Laffey JG, et al. Intubation practices and adverse peri-intubation events in critically ill patients from 29 countries. JAMA 2021;325: 1164–72.
8. Roth D, Pace NL, Lee A. Bedside tests for predicting difficult airways: An abridged Cochrane diagnostic test accuracy systematic review. Anaesthesia 2019;74:915–28.
9. Norskov AK, Rosenstock CV, Wettersley J, et al. Diagnostic accuracy of anaesthsiologists' prediction of difficulty airway management in daily clinical practice: a cohort study of 88,064 patients registered in the Danish Anaesthesia Database. Anaesthesia 2015;70:272–81.
10. Kornas RL, Owyang CG, Sakles JC, et al. Evaluation and management of the physiologically difficulty airway: Consensus recommendations from Society for Airway Management. Anesth Analg 2021;132:395–405.
11. Nimmagadda U, Salem MR, Crystal GJ. Preoxygenation: physiologic basis, benefitis, and potential risks. Anesth Analg 2017;124:507–17.

12. Berry CB, Myles PS. Preoxygenation in health volunteers: a graph of oxygen "washin" using end-tidal oxygraphy. Br J Anaesth 1994;72:116–8.
13. Campbell IT, Beatty PC. Monitoring preoxygenation. Br J Anaesth 1994;72:3–4.
14. Baraka AS, Taha SK, Aouad MT, et al. Preoxygenation: comparison of maximal breathing and tidal volume breathing techniques. Anesthsiology 1999;91:612–6.
15. Mosier JM, Hypes CD, Sakles JC. Understanding preoxygenation and apneic oxygenation during intubation in the critically ill. Intensive Care Med 2017;43: 226–8.
16. Wimalasena Y, Burns B, Reid C, et al. Apneic oxygenation was associated with decreased desaturation rates during rapid sequence intubation by an Australian helicopter emergency medicine service. Ann Emerg Med 2015;65:371–6.
17. Sakles JC, Mosier JM, Patanwala AE, et al. Apneic oxygenation is associated with a reduction in the incidence of hypoxemia during the RSI of patients with intracranial hemorrhage in the emergency department. Intern Emerg Med 2016;11(7): 983–92.
18. Casey JD, Janz DR, Russell DW, et al. Bag-mask ventilation during tracheal intubation of critically ill adults. N Engl J Med 2019;380:811–21.
19. Dixon BJ, Dixon JB, Carden JR, et al. Preoxygenation is more effective in the 25 degrees head-up position than in the supine position in severely obese patients: a randomized controlled study. Anesthsiology 2005;102:1110–5.
20. Smischney NJ. Evaluation of preintubation shock index and modified shock index as predictors of postintubation hypotension and other short-term outcomes. J Crit Care 2015;861:e1–7.
21. Rady MY, Rivers EP, Nowak RM. Resuscitation of the critically ill in the ED: responses of blood pressure, heart rate, shock index, central venous oxygen saturation, and lactate. Am J Emerg Med 1996;14:218–25.
22. Althunayyan SM. Shock index as a predictor of post-intubation hypotension and cardiac arrest; A review of the current evidence. Trauma 2019;7:21–7.
23. Heffner AC, Swords DS, Nussbaum ML, et al. Predictors of the complication of postintubation hypotension during emergency airway management. J Crit Care 2012;27:587–93.
24. Janz DR, Casey JD, Semler MW, et al. Effect of a fluid bolus on cardiovascular collapse among critically ill adults undergoing tracheal intubation (PrePARE): a randomized controlled trial. Lancet Respir Med 2019;7:1039–47.
25. Rotando A, Picard L, Delibert S, et al. Push dose pressors: experience in critically ill patients outside of the operating room. Am J Emerg Med 2019;37:494–8.
26. Cole JB, Knack SK, Karl ER, et al. Human errors and adverse hemodynamic events related to "push dose pressors" in the emergency department. J Med Toxicol 2019;15:276–86.
27. Smischney NJ, Kashyap R, Khanna AK, et al. Risk factors for and prediction of post-intubation hypotension in critically ill adults: a multicenter prospective cohort study. PLoS One 2020;15(8):e0233852.
28. Groetzinger LM, Williams J, Svec S, et al. Peripherally infused norepinephrine to avoid central venous catheter placement in a medical intensive care unit: a pilot study. Ann Pharmacother 2021;56(7):773–81. Online ahead of print.
29. Nguyen TT, Surrey A, Barmaan B, et al. Utilization and extravasation of peripheral norepinephrine in the emergency department. Am J Emerg Med 2021;39:55–9.
30. Tran QK, Mester G, Bzhilyanskaya V, et al. Complication of vasopressor infusion through peripheral venous catheter: a systematic review and meta-analysis. Am J Emerg Med 2020;38:2434–43.

31. Mosier JM, Joshi R, Hypes C, et al. The physiologically difficult airway. West J Emerg Med 2015;16:1109–17.
32. Whylock CW, Atkinson MS. Increasing use of an endotracheal intubation safety checklist in the emergency department. BMJ Open Qual 2021;10:e001575.
33. Forristal C, Hayman K, Smith N. Does utilization of an intubation safety checklist reduce omissions during simulated resuscitation scenarios: a multi-center randomized controlled trial. CJEM 2020;23:45.
34. Levin NM, Fix ML, April MD, et al. The association of rocuronium dosing and first-attempt intubation success in adult emergency department patients. CJEM 2021; 23:518–27.
35. Cook TM. Strategies for the prevention of airway complications – a narrative review. Anaesthesia 2018;73:93–111.
36. Alhomary M, Ramadan E, Curran E, et al. Videolaryngoscopy vs. fiberoptic bronchoscopy for awake tracheal intubation: a systematic review and meta-analysis. Anaesthesia 2018;73:1151–61.
37. Law JA, Morris IR, Brousseau PA, et al. The incidence, success rate, and complications of awake tracheal intubaton in 1,554 patients over 12 years: a historical cohort study. Can J Anesth 2015;62:736–44.
38. Joseph TT, Gal JS, DeMaria SJ, et al. A retrospective study of success, failure, and time needed to perform awake intubation. Anesthesiology 2016;125:105–14.
39. Cho EA, Hwang SH, Lee SH, et al. Does glycopyrrolate premedication facilitate tracheal intubation with a rigid video-stylet? A randomized controlled trial. Medicine 2018;97:e11834.
40. El-Boghdadly K, Pawa A, Chin KJ. Local anesthetic systemic toxicity: current prospectives. Local Reg Anesth 2018;11:35–44.
41. Xue FS, Liu HP, He N, et al. Spray-as-you-go airway topical anesthesia in patients with a difficult airway: a randomized, double-blind comparison of 2% and 4% lidocaine. Anesth Analg 2009;108:536–43.
42. Baekgaard JS, Eskesen TG, Sillesen M, et al. Ketamine as a rapid sequence induction agent in the trauma population: A systematic review. Anesth Analg 2019; 128:504–10.
43. Kramer N, Lebowitz D, Walsh M. Rapid sequence intubation in traumatic brain-injured adult. Cureus 2018;10:e2530.
44. Bar-Joseph G, Guilburd Y, Tamir A, et al. Effectiveness of ketamine in decreasing intracranial pressure in children with intracranial hypertension. J Neurosurg Pediatr 2009;4:40–6.
45. Pantawala AE, Erstad BL, Roe DJ, et al. Succinylcholine is associated with increased mortality when used for rapid sequence intubation of severe brain injured patients in the emergency department. Pharmacotherapy 2016;36:57–63.

Moving?

Make sure your subscription moves with you!

To notify us of your new address, find your **Clinics Account Number** (located on your mailing label above your name), and contact customer service at:

Email: journalscustomerservice-usa@elsevier.com

800-654-2452 (subscribers in the U.S. & Canada)
314-447-8871 (subscribers outside of the U.S. & Canada)

Fax number: 314-447-8029

Elsevier Health Sciences Division
Subscription Customer Service
3251 Riverport Lane
Maryland Heights, MO 63043

*To ensure uninterrupted delivery of your subscription, please notify us at least 4 weeks in advance of move.

Printed and bound by CPI Group (UK) Ltd, Croydon, CR0 4YY

08/05/2025

01864723-0011